Critical Care Outreach

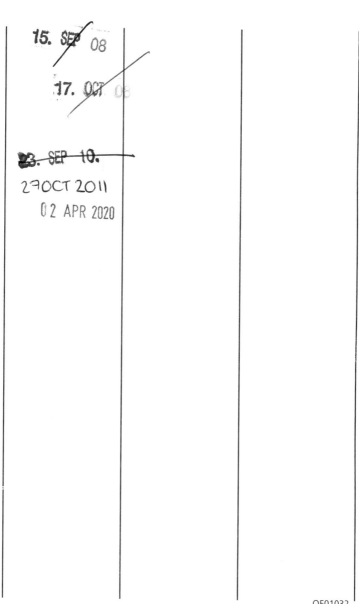

Critical Care Outreach

Edited by

LEE R CUTLER RN, BSC (HONS), MA (ED)

WAYNE P ROBSON RN, BMEDSCI (HONS), MSC (CRIT CARE)

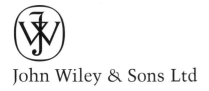

John Wiley & Sons Ltd

Other Wiley Editorial Offices

John Wiley & Sons Inc., 111 River Street, Hoboken, NJ 07030, USA

Jossey-Bass, 989 Market Street, San Francisco, CA 94103-1741, USA

Wiley-VCH Verlag GmbH, Boschstr. 12, D-69469 Weinheim, Germany

John Wiley & Sons Australia Ltd, 42 McDougall Street, Milton, Queensland 4064, Australia

John Wiley & Sons (Asia) Pte Ltd, 2 Clementi Loop #02-01, Jin Xing Distripark, Singapore 129809

John Wiley & Sons Canada Ltd, 6045 Freemont Blvd, Mississauga, ONT, L5R 4J3

Wiley also publishes its books in a variety of electronic formats. Some content that appears in print may not be available in electronic books.

Library of Congress Cataloging-in-Publication Data

Critical care outreach / edited by Lee R. Cutler, Wayne P. Robson.
    p. ; cm.
Includes bibliographical references and index.
ISBN-13: 978-0-470-02584-0 (pbk. : alk. paper)
ISBN-10: 0-470-02584-0 (pbk. : alk. paper)
 1. Intensive care nursing – Great Britain.   I. Cutler, Lee R.   II. Robson, Wayne P.
 [DNLM: 1. Critical Care – methods – Great Britain.   2. Critical Care – organization & administration – Great Britain.   3. Community-Institutional Relations – Great Britain.   4. Intensive Care Units – organization & administration – Great Britain.
5. Patient Care Team – organization & administration – Great Britain.
WX 218 C93636 2006]
RT120.I5C75 2006
616.02'8 – dc22
                                                                              2006001111

British Library Cataloguing in Publication Data

A catalogue record for this book is available from the British Library
ISBN-13 978-0-470-02584-0
ISBN-10 0-470-02584-0

Typeset by SNP Best-set Typesetter Ltd., Hong Kong
Printed and bound in Great Britain by TJ International Ltd, Padstow, Cornwall
This book is printed on acid-free paper responsibly manufactured from sustainable forestry in which at least two trees are planted for each one used for paper production.

Contents

List of contributors

EDITORS

Lee R Cutler RN, BSc (Hons), MA (Ed)

Lee is a consultant nurse in critical care at Doncaster and Bassetlaw Hospitals NHS Foundation Trust and honorary senior lecturer at the University of Sheffield. He has practised, taught, researched and published in the field of critical care for over a decade. He qualified as a nurse in 1992 and since then has worked in Rotherham, Leeds, Sheffield, Doncaster and Bassetlaw in clinical and academic posts in critical care. He gained a BSc (Hons) in Nursing at the University of Hull and an MA in Education at the University of Sheffield. At 30 he became one of the youngest consultant nurses and has been in post now for five years leading the nursing contribution to critical care outreach within Doncaster and Bassetlaw Hospitals.

Wayne P Robson RN, BMedSci (Hons), MSc (Crit Care)

Wayne trained at Manchester Royal Infirmary, and has worked within the field of critical care for the past 14 years, in intensive care, coronary care and high dependency in a variety of posts including charge nurse on HDU, and a critical care outreach nurse. Wayne helped set up the critical care outreach service at the Royal Hallamshire Hospital in Sheffield. He is currently the nurse consultant in critical care at Chesterfield Royal Hospital NHS Foundation Trust, and is an honorary lecturer at the University of Sheffield. He leads the critical care outreach team at Chesterfield Royal Hospital. He has published a number of articles on sepsis, critical care outreach, and the physical after effects of intensive care, and has presented papers at national and international critical care conferences. Wayne led the introduction of patient diaries onto intensive care, and has a special interest in how patients make sense of their ITU experience. He is a passionate supporter of the Surviving Sepsis Campaign and promoting early recognition and management of patients with severe sepsis.

CONTRIBUTORS

Derek Bainbridge PgCert, BA (Hons), DipN, RGN, ENB 100, 405
Derek has worked in critical care since 1979. He was senior nurse at Rotherham General Hospital from 1991 before being appointed nurse consultant in 2002. Derek was also lead nurse for the North Trent Critical Care Network and helped to develop outreach teams both locally and regionally.

Kate Bray MSc, BA (Hons), RGN
Kate trained at University College Hospital London, and moved to Sheffield in 1984. She has held posts of clinical educator, and practice development nurse in critical care and is currently the nurse consultant in critical care for Sheffield Teaching Hospitals NHS Foundation Trust. In June 2001 Kate joined the National Board of the British Association of Critical Care Nurses (BACCN) as professional adviser.

Judith M Cutler RN, DipN, Dip Crit Care, BA (Hons), PGDipEd
Judith is a clinical nurse educator in critical care at Doncaster and Bassetlaw Hospitals NHS Foundation Trust. She has been in post for over four years and has worked in critical care for 10 years.

Professor David L. Edbrooke LRCP, MRCS, MRCOG, FFARCS
David has been a clinician in intensive care for 25 years. He is professor of intensive care medicine at Sheffield Hallam University, and director of the Medical Economics and Research Centre Sheffield (MERCS). He has written approximately 100 peer reviewed publications, and has delivered approximately 100 invited lectures worldwide.

Dr Jeremy Groves MBBS, FRCA
Jeremy has been a consultant anaesthetist on intensive care at Chesterfield Royal Hospital NHS Foundation Trust for 10 years. He has played a major role in establishing and developing the Trust's critical care outreach team.

Denise Honnor RGN, ENB 100, 998
Denise is currently senior sister in the critical care outreach team at Doncaster and Bassetlaw Hospitals NHS Foundation Trust. She trained at Doncaster and has worked in intensive care, general and specialist surgical nurse posts. She has worked in critical care for over 20 years.

Rinky Inglis RGN, ENB N53, 100
Rinky is a critical care outreach sister at Sheffield Teaching Hospitals NHS Foundation Trust, and was a founder member of the critical care outreach team at the Northern General Hospital site.

Sally Knightly BSc (Hons) Physiotherapy

Sally qualified in 1991 and after becoming a senior II physiotherapist she specialised in respiratory care. In 1995 she became the senior I physiotherapist with responsibility for intensive care. Since 2001 she has worked as an outreach practitioner with the critical care outreach team at the Royal Oldham Hospital.

Alex Larkin MSc, RGN

Alex has worked in the field of critical care nursing and resuscitation training since qualifying in 1988. Alex currently works as a nurse consultant in critical care and is responsible for the implementation and development of the critical care outreach service within one of the sites at the Pennine Acute Hospitals NHS Trusts.

Denise Penney RGN, ENB 100

Denise is a senior sister on the intensive care unit at Chesterfield Royal Hospital NHS Foundation Trust. She helped introduce patient diaries onto intensive care. Her special interests include renal failure and CVVH, teaching and staff development.

Nicola Platts BSc(Hons), MPhil

Since joining the NHS 1996 Nicola has held a series of change management posts where she has had exposure to facilitating small-scale local service improvement projects and involvement in large-scale Trust projects including merger processes. Nicola is currently a service improvement manager at Sheffield Teaching Hospitals NHS Trust where she provides practical support and advice to multidisciplinary teams to redesign processes and adopt new ways of working. Nicola also draws from experiences as the lead for service improvement for the North Trent Critical Care Network, which was part of the Modernisation Agency Critical Care Programme between 2001 and 2004.

Elaine Shaw RGN, ENB100, ENB 998

Elaine is currently senior sister with the critical care outreach team at Doncaster and Bassetlaw Hospitals NHS Foundation Trust. She trained in Doncaster and has worked in critical care for over 20 years.

Sue Shepherd MSc, PSM

Sue is currently network manager for Mid-Trent Critical Care Network, and is responsible for overseeing service improvement within the network. Sue has a real passion for service improvement and works with front line staff to facilitate changes and improvements in service delivery. In 2003 she completed her MSc in public services management and her thesis examined the effectiveness of process redesign training in critical care and explored clinicians' resistance to change. Sue continues to provide process redesign training to individuals and groups within and outside the network.

Jayne Tague RGN, ENB 100, ENB N53
Jayne has extensive experience in both critical care and surgery, and was a founder member of the critical care outreach team at Chesterfield Royal Hospital. After five years as a senior sister with the outreach team, Jayne is now a matron for the Medical Directorate.

Kathryn Warren BA (Hons), DipN, RGN, ENB100
Kathryn is a critical care outreach sister at Sheffield Teaching Hospitals NHS Foundation Trust, and was a founder member of the critical care outreach team at the Northern General Hospital site. She is currently acting as lead nurse for the North Trent Critical Care Network.

Gayle Wheeldon RGN, ENB 100
Gayle is a sister on the intensive care unit at Chesterfield Royal Hospital NHS Foundation Trust and helped to introduce patient diaries onto intensive care.

Dr Paul Whiting MBChB, FRCA
Paul is currently a specialist registrar (Spr) in anaesthetics, and has an interest in intensive care and critical care outreach.

Dr David Wood MBBS, FRCA
David is the lead consultant for critical care services including outreach for Doncaster and Bassetlaw NHS Foundation Trust. He has been involved in the development of the Trust's outreach team since 2000.

I The Evolution of Critical Care Outreach

1 The origins of critical care outreach

DEREK BAINBRIDGE

INTRODUCTION

The purpose of this chapter is to provide the reader with background information into the establishment of outreach services within the United Kingdom (UK). The chapter will identify and explain the political drivers, and will discuss key documents that recommended the development of outreach and government proposals. International examples of outreach will be discussed alongside the development of outreach services within the UK, highlighting evidence around sub-optimal care and the need for early intervention.

DEVELOPMENT OF A NEW SERVICE

Critical care outreach teams were developed in England as a direct result of the Audit Commission's report, *Critical to Success*, published in 1999 (Audit Commission 1999) and the Department of Health's publication *Comprehensive Critical Care: A Review of Adult Critical Care Services* (DoH 2000). *Comprehensive Critical Care* was a key document developed by a multi-professional group of experts drawn from a number of eminent clinicians in critical care, organisations affiliated to critical care such as the Intensive Care Society, Royal Colleges and senior health service managers. The expert group was established by the Department of Health in March 1999 to propose a framework for the future organisation and delivery of adult critical care services in England that was evidence based and fitted into the modernisation agenda.

The expert group's vision for the future of critical care services in England included the establishment of an outreach team to provide and support the care of critically ill patients, or those at risk of becoming critically ill on general wards. The expert group also recommended that the service needed to be set within an effective whole hospital bed management system, which ensured that every patient was in an appropriate location to meet their needs for staffing and equipment to support their care.

Critical Care Outreach. Edited by Lee Cutler and Wayne Robson.
Copyright 2006 by John Wiley & Sons Ltd.

The development of critical care networks was also a key organisational factor that supported and encouraged the development of the critical care outreach service as part of the health improvement programme. In the spring of 2000 the Department of Health held workshops in the eight NHS regions. Regional offices were encouraged to work with NHS trusts to form clinical networks. Representatives from all intensive care units, higher education providers, commissioners and other stakeholders met with regional leads to test the extent of multi-disciplinary support and cooperation for the proposals outlined in *Comprehensive Critical Care.*

Some of the earlier networks already had traditional associations either through the geography, links with academic institutions or the existing training rotations for medical staff. The objective for the development of networks was for neighbouring NHS trust hospitals to work together to meet the needs of all critically ill patients in their geographical area. This working together not only involved the providers but also, importantly, the commissioners of critical care services. Commissioners were responsible for assessing need and ensuring that appropriate resources were available to develop the recommendations set out in *Comprehensive Critical Care.*

Trent Regional Health Authority was one of the first regions to develop critical care networks, splitting the region into three: North Trent, Mid Trent and South Trent. Trent Regional office already had an intensive care lead in post, who was also a member of the expert group, to coordinate and organise regional meetings. Trent Region was arguably a pioneer of the network concept and, through vision, commitment, enthusiasm and drive, Trent developed three networks early in June 2000, appointing a full-time network manager, clinical and nursing leads for each network. Each network within Trent Region appointed a chair and steering group as well as the management team. The steering group consisted of senior doctors, nurses and managers whose role was to discuss the implementation of the proposals, and to prioritise developments and secure the funding available centrally.

The networks would meet with the regional offices' intensive care lead to discuss how the service requirements would be funded and performance managed. Trent Region managed the £14,709,000 allocated to it from within the £150 million for critical care services throughout England. In comparison the London region received £23,409,000 (DoH Health Service Circular 2000/16, winter 2000/01).

The allocation of additional resources for critical care was on the basis of weighted capitation allowing all regions to develop critical care services. Allocations were made to regional offices rather than directly to the health authorities. Regional offices nationally were then expected to work with local health communities to ensure that the resources were used effectively to build in capacity for the winter but also to assist with the modernisation of the service over the coming years. Regional offices were to submit plans which were analysed to ensure that they represented effective use of the additional resources and that they achieved increased capacity and made progress with the modernisation agenda.

Another crucial development that assisted the outreach team was the Critical Care Modernisation Programme led by the National Patient Access Team. This team was established to oversee the modernisation of critical care services in particular supporting service redesign. The National Patient Access Team later became the Modernisation Agency's Critical Care Programme in 2002, which then further developed the network concept incorporating service redesign, process mapping and PDSA (Plan Do Study Act) as a tool to effect change. The involvement of the Modernisation Agency in networks was essential, otherwise the momentum and standardisation across the UK would have been lost, and more health communities would not have benefited from the network concept and the service improvement agenda. However, not all regional offices and NHS trusts within England were as enthusiastic and committed to the network concept of working together as Trent was. Indeed not all of the monies allocated to regional offices went into the development of critical care services, which may have contributed to the differences in developments nationally.

ROLE OF CRITICAL CARE OUTREACH

The role of the outreach service is primarily to ensure that critically ill patients, or those at risk of becoming so, receive appropriate and timely treatment in the most suitable location within the hospital environment. In the UK these new services were called 'outreach', implying an extension or reaching out of the usual critical care service provided. However, other titles exist such as the Medical Emergency Team (MET), the Patient At Risk Team (PART) and the postoperative care team. However, the development and concept of an outreach team is not new. The concept of an outreach team was first developed in Liverpool, New South Wales, Australia, in 1990 with the development of the Medical Emergency Team (MET). The MET replaced the traditional cardiac arrest team by adopting a more proactive approach and the development of a scoring system to identify those patients at risk of impending critical illness and therefore early intervention in an attempt to improve outcome (Lee et al. 1995). Extending the role of the cardiac arrest team acknowledges the fact that cardiac arrests are commonly preceded by premonitory signs and symptoms (Franklin and Mathew 1994).

The MET has much in common with the shock trauma teams first described by Frank (1967). Evidence suggests that earlier intervention, active management and earlier admission to intensive care may have some benefit to the patient in terms of outcome if treatment is initiated early (Goldhill et al. 1999).

Frequently patients are admitted to the intensive care unit following cardiac arrest on the ward with little or no hope of survival. Evidence exists that suggests that most of these patients have deranged physiology prior to the cardiac arrest and that failure to recognise critically ill patients on the ward results in a death that potentially could have been prevented (Dubois and Brook 1988). Physiological deterioration prior to cardio-respiratory arrest is either therefore not recognised or inadequately treated.

Respiratory rate, heart rate and oxygenation have all been highlighted as indicators of pending critical illness, but unfortunately the monitoring and charting of physiological variables, especially respiratory rate, is often poor. This omission of respiratory rate, one of the most sensitive triggers, has been shown to be mainly due to the use of mechanical devices for recording blood pressure, heart rate and pulse oximetry. Sadly the machines don't record respiratory rate and therefore this observation is often omitted from the set of observations. These claims have been more recently studied; Buist et al. (2002) and Bellomo et al. (2003) concluded in two separate studies that in clinically unstable inpatients early intervention by a medical emergency team significantly reduced the incidence of and mortality from unexpected cardiac arrest.

Other drivers for change and improvement of service delivery existed within the UK, which highlighted deficits in the quality of care before admission to intensive care. During the past decade deficiencies in the quality of medical care have precipitated detailed scrutiny in the form of national confidential inquiries. As early as 1993 the National Confidential Enquiry into Perioperative Deaths (NCEPOD) highlighted deficiencies in postoperative management of patients. The report showed that two-thirds of deaths following surgery occurred three or more days after surgery on the ward, usually as a result of cardio-respiratory complications, renal failure, or infection (NCEPOD 1996). The report also identified a 'substantial shortfall in critical care services', particularly High Dependency Unit provision nationally.

Sub-optimal care patients received prior to admission to intensive care also raised concern by some authors. McQuillan in a confidential inquiry identified that of 100 patients studied 54 received sub-optimal care prior to admission and that the mortality of these patients was 48%, almost twice that of the 20 that had been treated appropriately. In addition to poor management the inquiry highlighted that two-thirds of the 54 patients were admitted late to intensive care (McQuillan et al. 1998).

Issues around sub-optimal care are not unique to the UK. The Harvard Medical Practice Study 1 (Brennan et al. 1991) randomly reviewed 30,121 patient records from 51 randomly selected acute hospitals in New York State in 1984. It concluded that there is a substantial amount of injury to patients from medical management, and many injuries are the result of substandard care.

EDUCATION AND SUPPORT

Supporting staff on the wards is a key component of outreach teams, but this concept is not new: as early as 1999 Coad described the role of the critical care nurse supporting ward staff in the care of critically ill patients outside the critical care unit (Coad and Haines 1999). Indeed the Audit Commission's study demonstrated some interesting findings that support this. The study reported that 94% of the 243 units responding stated that critical care nurses visited wards to advise on specialist areas of care, while on 70% of the units' critical care nurses visited wards to liaise regarding the admission and/ or discharge of patients. Therefore, the concept of intensive care nurses supporting ward staff is not totally new and the criticism of intensive care staff and units being removed, remote and inaccessible may be unjustified in some hospitals. However, it could be argued that many intensive care units within hospitals are not unlike 'nuclear bunkers', due to the design, access and mystique that surround the intensive care unit. Modernisation, service redesign and development of outreach teams have broken down and will continue to break down many barriers in the development of a hospital-wide systematic approach to care.

As a result of the Audit Commission's recommendations the development of critical care outreach teams became one of the key objectives discussed in *Comprehensive Critical Care: A Review of Adult Critical Care Services* (1999) published by the Department of Health (2000). Since the introduction of outreach teams within the UK, a number of models and titles have evolved. However, the principles largely remain the same following the model first described within *Comprehensive Critical Care*. Whichever model is chosen to develop locally, outreach should form part of a coordinated approach to the support of all patients with a need for critical care. This concept is underpinned by the belief that all those patients deemed to be at risk are entitled to an appropriate referral, timely management and nursing care wherever they are within the hospital.

Critical care outreach services have three essential objectives:

1. to avert admission;
2. to enable discharge;
3. to share critical care skills.

The establishment of outreach services within the UK differs from that of the MET inasmuch as outreach teams are primarily seen as providing support for staff, averting admission, ensuring more timely admission and enabling discharge of patients from critical care.

However, the model adopted by each hospital should be established to address the specific issues and type of service required by them; therefore some outreach teams will be more interventionist than others and therefore mirror medical emergency management teams.

Many reasons exist nationally pointing to why the hospital system is occasionally failing. Inadequate nurse staffing levels on the wards may lead to failure to recognise the sick ward patient due to skill mix, experience and knowledge. The diploma style nurse training has always received much criticism, as it has been seen to reduce the clinical skills of newly qualified nurses due to the change in the curriculum.

Nurses are not solely to blame for sub-optimal care. Inexperienced medical staff may not respond to the deteriorating patient appropriately or quickly enough. Changes brought about by the Calman reforms (1994) have led to a shortened training programme and more cross covering of specialties particularly in medicine. Training is a key area of concern: undergraduate and postgraduate training does not address the specific training and skills required to manage the deteriorating sick ward patient.

Demographic and case mix changes within the hospital population have made the patient population older and sicker. The wards are no longer diluted with the young short stay cases since the advent of dedicated day surgery units. Many of the inpatient services are becoming specialised, resulting in the deskilling of ward staff.

Having highlighted the possible problems, which have contributed to suboptimal care, it is very important that hospital managers don't see outreach teams as a substitute for insufficient intensive and high dependency beds, inadequate ward staffing, inexperienced trainees, lack of senior medical supervision or inappropriate skill mix. Neither should the outreach team assume the clinical responsibility for the care of all patients at risk of critical illness from other departments within the hospital.

POLITICAL DRIVERS

Media coverage in the late 1990s and early 2000 highlighted the shortage of intensive care beds. The incoming Labour Government in 1997 admitted that there had been a lack of investment in critical care capacity, leading to pressure on the system particularly during the winter period. This shortage became national news, mainly because patients requiring critical care were either being transferred elsewhere or were dying. Media headlines such as 'Vital surgery cancelled seven times' (BBC News 2000), 'Intensive care beds run out' (BBC News 1999), 'NHS crisis as flu grips Britain' (Wintour et al. 2000) became everyday headlines. NHS hospitals were reporting shortages in intensive care beds as a result of the elderly becoming critically ill and requiring intensive care, the problem in many hospitals being exacerbated by staff falling ill as well. The flu outbreak in 2000 stretched many hospitals to breaking point and led to an acute shortage of intensive care beds. Liam Donaldson, chief medical officer, revealed in a press statement that there were probably twice as many people suffering from flu as official figures suggested, and declared, 'it is a serious flu epidemic'.

Issues around the transferring of patients long distances became headlines due to the acute shortage of intensive care beds. Private hospitals had offered to help ease the intensive care bed crisis by leasing beds to the NHS, an idea backed by the Tory Health spokesperson Dr Liam Fox. But Health Secretary Alan Milburn insisted that the NHS was coping, and said that any patient who needed intensive care would receive it. There were even plans for some patients to be sent to France for treatment if required (Wintour et al. 2000).

Clearly there was a crisis within the NHS due to capacity and demand issues. However, issues around planning and the organisation of health care became a priority as the flu epidemic hit planned admissions and necessitated the cancellation of elective patients and the transfer of the critically ill. Ambulances transferring critically ill patients often passed intensive care units with an empty bed, anecdotal evidence suggests that some intensive care units would declare themselves being full when clearly they had a bed. This occurred due to lack of organisation and protectionism of local critical care beds.

Comprehensive Critical Care aimed to deliver a service systematically across the whole health system by modernisation, the development of networks, a planned approach to workforce development, developing a culture of data collection and an integrated hospital-wide approach, with the development of services which extend beyond the physical boundaries of intensive care such as critical care outreach.

The government stated within the publication of the NHS Plan that there would be a 30% increase in adult critical care beds to address the shortfall. However, more significantly the government published the report *Comprehensive Critical Care* (DoH 2000) that looked at changing the way in which critical care was delivered. The term 'without walls' was phrased by the National Patient Access Team (which later became the Modernisation Agency): rather than providing intensive and high dependency beds, the service should be 'without walls' and based on illness severity.

In March 1999 there were 1520 intensive care beds and 720 high dependency beds; by January 2004 this had risen to 1769 and 1374 respectively (see Table 1.1).

Comprehensive Critical Care was a key document in the development of critical care outreach teams nationally. Never before had a service been recommended in a government document without any evidence that the service would deliver efficiencies, economy and effectiveness.

As a result of media pressure, the publication of the Audit Commission's report and *Comprehensive Critical Care* the Government announced in May 2000 a massive shake-up of NHS critical care services. As an unprecedented acknowledgement, Alan Milburn, the then Secretary of State for Health, announced that he was accepting in full all the recommendations drawn up by the expert group within *Comprehensive Critical Care*.

Critical care outreach suddenly became a reality for many working within critical care; £150 million had been allocated to implement all the reforms identified within *Comprehensive Critical Care*. A priority for regional offices was the development of 50 outreach teams nationally by the winter of 2001.

Table 1.1 Number of critical care beds on census day

Census date	Intensive care	High dependency	Total
31 March 1999	1520	720	2240
30 September 1999	1501	740	2241
15 January 2000	1555	807	2362
14 July 2000	1496	847	2343
15 January 2001	1677	1208	2885
16 July 2001	1670	1270	2940
15 January 2002	1711	1319	3030
16 July 2002	1718	1352	3070
15 January 2003	1746	1351	3097
16 July 2003	1731	1397	3128
15 January 2004	1769	1374	3143

Source: Department of Health form KH03a.

Indeed by August 2000, 65 outreach teams had been set up which prompted Lord Hunt to say that 'the outreach teams signal a sea change in critical care'.

Critical care outreach has continued to develop. In a speech delivered by Rosie Winterton, MP, Health Minister to the NHS Modernisation Agency sharing event in March 2004, she identified that there were now 170 critical care outreach teams out of a total of 220 acute hospitals with critical care services, and that the government would like to see an outreach team in every hospital (DoH 2004).

REFERENCES

Audit Commission (1999) *Critical to Success: The Place of Efficient and Effective Critical Care Services within the Acute Hospital.* London: Audit Commission.

BBC News (1999) Intensive care beds run out, Thursday, 7 January. http://www.bbc.co.uk/1/hi/health/250008.stm

BBC News (2000) Vital surgery cancelled seven times, Monday, 17 January. http://www.bbc.co.uk/1/hi/health/607538.stm

Bellomo R, Goldsmith D, Uchino S (2003) A prospective before and after trial of a medical emergency team. *The Medical Journal of Australia* 179(6): 283–7.

Brennan TA, Leape LL, Laird NM (1991) Incidence of adverse events and negligence in hospitalised patients. Results of the Harvard Medical Practice Study 1. *The New England Journal of Medicine* 324(6): 370–6.

Buist MD, Moore GE, Bernard SA (2002) Effects of a medical emergency team on reduction of incidence of and mortality from unexpected cardiac arrest in hospital. *British Medical Journal* 324: 387–90.

Coad S, Haines S (1999) Supporting staff caring for critically ill patients in acute areas. *Nursing in Critical Care* 4: 245–8.

Department of Health (2000) *Comprehensive Critical Care: A Review of Adult Critical Care Services.* London: Department of Health.

Dubois RW, Brook RH (1988) Preventable deaths: who, how often and why? *Annals of Internal Medicine* 109: 582–9.

Frank ED (1967) A shock team in a general hospital. *Anesthesia and Analgesia* 46: 740–5.

Franklin C, Mathew J (1994) Developing strategies to prevent in hospital cardiac arrest: analysing responses of physicians and nurses in the hours before the event. *Critical Care Medicine* 22: 244–7.

Goldhill DR, Worthington L, Mulcahy A et al. (1999) The patient at risk team: identifying and managing seriously ill ward patients. *Anaesthesia* 54: 853–60.

Lee A, Bishop G, Hillman KM, Daffurn K (1995) The medical emergency team. *Anaesthesia and Intensive Care* 23: 183–6.

McQuillan P, Pilkington S, Allan A (1998) Confidential inquiry into quality of care before admission to intensive care. *British Medical Journal* 316: 1853–8.

Moore E (2000) Getting the bug. *Observer,* 18 January. www.guardian.co.uk/guardianeducation/story

NCEPOD (1993) *National Confidential Enquiry into Perioperative Deaths.* London: HMSO.

NCEPOD (1996) *National Confidential Enquiry into Perioperative Deaths.* London: HMSO.

Wintour P, McVeigh T, Browne A (2000) NHS crisis as flu grips Britain. *Observer,* 9 January. http://search.guardian.co.uk

2 Designing an outreach service

DAVID WOOD

INTRODUCTION

The concept of critical care outreach developed in response to a range of identified deficiencies in the management of patients during the early phases of an acute severe illness. These have been well documented in the wider literature and summaries are provided within this text (see for example, Chapters 1 and 5). The underlying principles of outreach are to identify patients who are critically ill, or are at risk of becoming so, and then to improve their management by paying particular attention to the basics of physiological support. Every hospital will have a different pattern of deficiencies and different critical care service configurations. The types of changes that will be required and the relative importance of each change will determine the challenges faced by a fledgling outreach team. A structuring of the priorities of the service can only be decided after careful assessment of the systems currently in place. This chapter will discuss a number of areas that need to be considered when designing a critical care outreach team and describe a process that will lead to an adaptable team evolving to meet the specific needs of its hospital and is intended for those developing an outreach service or redesigning their team.

DESIGN ISSUES

When planning an outreach service a number of distinct but interacting factors need to be considered. These factors include the team composition and size as well as organisational issues such as the intended team methodology, hours of cover and communication strategy. Improving any aspect of health care involves a degree of change being made to the current system. The team will inevitably be the catalyst for change and so the design of the team will need to be tailored to the specific challenges that the team will face.

In order to allow informed decisions to be made it is essential to understand the nature and scale of the issues to be faced. Once the nature and scale of the problem are understood it becomes possible to assess the advantages and

Critical Care Outreach. Edited by Lee Cutler and Wayne Robson.
Copyright 2006 by John Wiley & Sons Ltd.

disadvantages of each factor of the team design. Once the design is optimised then the strategy for introducing the service needs to be considered.

Recognising that the team may have been designed incorrectly, or that an unforeseen challenge will prevent the team from achieving its goals, can be very difficult. A new service introduced to address problems will only succeed if it is prepared to accept that it will need to evolve and change. Continuous re-evaluation of the problems the team faces as well as the team's approach will inform changes in methodology or process redesign.

ASSESSING DEFICIENCIES IN THE CURRENT SYSTEM

A key principle that should be employed when undertaking any initiative of a problem-solving nature is first to seek to understand the problem fully before you set about designing the solution, or selecting from a range of options. This is fundamental; however, it is extremely common to see people driving forward their vision of what the solution should be without a thorough understanding of the problem – its nature, extent, causes or contributing factors as well as having a range of anecdotes and examples that can help communicate these to others.

These principles are communicated in two maxims; first Covey (1989) asserts that one should always 'Seek first to understand ... then to be understood'.

Secondly, as an eminently wise colleague of mine once said, 'It takes a wealth of experience to realise that the most important things are the basics.' Success usually involves getting these right first and then moving on to the more complex things. In the following few paragraphs I have attempted to give a flavour of the understanding we came to and the implications for outreach.

Probably the simplest way to start to identify deficiencies in the current system is to hold a number of informal 'discovery' interviews with clinical staff throughout the hospital. This type of relatively informal probing is generally very effective at identifying the potential range of problems. It elicits a series of anecdotes and examples that can be followed up and learned from. However my experience is that any solution proposed during the interview must be subjected to rigorous analysis before being allowed to influence the planned development of the team. Otherwise it might simply be putting the solution before an understanding of the problem.

A number of more detailed audit projects may be useful to identify the scale and severity of the system defects. These audit projects can also be repeated once the outreach team is running to identify team successes. This type of quantitative audit may include: frequency of cardiac arrest calls, severity of sickness scoring of patients admitted to ICU or HDU from the wards, and readmission rates for patients discharged from ICU. Once a list of 'failings' has been compiled then the root causes need to be identified. These root causes can be very difficult to identify as a panoply of justifications, excuses and plausible reasons why the current system is the only possible one often hides them. We were not alone in finding delayed referrals to ICU and undetected deterioration as well as failures in care. These were ubiquitous throughout acute care areas in the NHS and unfortunately persist to some extent despite outreach (NCEPOD 2005).

In my experience the systems for identifying and treating critically ill patients fail for a number of reasons. These include: failure to recognise the severity of illness and to manage the problem appropriately; failure of staff to call appropriately skilled help until it is too late; and inadequate facilities for the delivery of higher levels of care.

Identifying a critically ill patient requires the ability to detect signs that the disease process has affected the patient's physiology to such an extent that vital organs are about to fail. There are a number of reasons for failure to make this assessment correctly, which we discovered through closely observing and process mapping the practice of observation rounds in ward areas.

Staff may be inadequately trained, or they may even be incorrectly trained so that they assume that signs of deterioration are not significant. The pressure to delegate basic nursing tasks such as observation rounds to less qualified personnel may result in personnel who are unable to process the results of their actions (unless also empowered and encouraged to do so).

Separating the task of collecting information from the process of analysing the information creates the potential for loss or corruption of the data before it can be processed. The goal of collecting the data rather than interpreting and reporting it, if abnormal, may be a priority in a culture of task allocation and 'getting the work done'. There is then potential for significant delay in recognition of the severity or urgency of a situation. Previously healthy patients with good physiological reserves may compensate so well for a severe physiological deficit that the severity of their illness is not recognised until the compensatory mechanisms fail and the patient collapses. A classic example of this type of problem is the young fit patient with pneumonia who appears to be coping with the illness for several days until they suddenly have a cardiac arrest. Reviewing the observation chart it becomes apparent that the patient will have been tachypnoeic, tachycardic and oliguric for a significant period before the collapse. Inadequacies in clinical observations and associated care as a response to physiological aberration have long been documented in the literature and continue to be a problem (NCEPOD 2005).

The implications for outreach service design are that the culture and practice of making, recording, reporting and acting on basic clinical observations have to be changed. Observations need to be seen as important and valued. This is an example of the 'what' – the goals and priorities for outreach. The 'how' is another matter, one which is more likely to divide opinion and for which local solutions are needed.

Staff inadequately trained to manage the situation may also be a problem, as was the case in our hospital. Training and education in the principles of managing critically ill patients for undergraduates, as well as more experienced and senior professionals, have in the past been woefully inadequate (DoH 2000; Goldacre et al. 2003). Clearly again there is an implication here about 'what' needs to be addressed. 'How' this can be achieved is the focus of Chapter 5 since outreach teams are ideally placed to provide a link between this type of training and its application at a ward level.

Doctors and nurses are often uncomfortable with asking for senior help, possibly because they feel that needing assistance is a sign of inadequacy. There is also a strong tradition of accepting that an immediate superior is the gatekeeper for access to more senior or the most appropriate source of advice or support. Ward-based staff may also delay calling for critical care advice or support because they do not feel that the patient is 'ill enough yet'. Instead they opt to continue to struggle to treat the patient, thus effectively waiting until the patient has deteriorated to a point where avoiding prolonged critical care treatment is no longer possible.

The implication for outreach design and priority setting is to change how and when healthcare professionals ask others for help when they are concerned about a patient. This is a further example of 'what' outreach has to address. The 'how' takes us into a debate over whether educative–supportive or interventionist models of outreach are best. This is dealt with a little later.

A further example of the issues to consider here is the capacity for the delivery of higher level care. It is a commonly held belief that managing critically ill patients requires specialist technical equipment and monitoring. The deficiencies in treatment prompting the development of outreach services were basically the appropriate administration of oxygen and fluids, neither of which requires specialist equipment. However, if the hospital has an inadequate provision of Level 2 (HDU) and Level 3 (ICU) beds then appropriate delivery of higher level care will be adversely affected, and the outreach team may need to be large enough to support the temporary provision of Level 2 or 3 care on a ward. Thus we are back to 'what' outreach should address. In this case it may be to take critical care to the ward (in the short term) rather than taking the ward patient to the ICU. These issues are highly political and should be discussed at the highest levels within the hospital. Nevertheless they are about 'what' outreach will inevitably become involved in and 'how' the team deals with it.

A final example of 'what' is essential work for outreach is to identify areas of strength within the current system. These may include particularly enthusiastic or influential ward sisters, physicians or surgeons who think outreach is a good idea and who want to influence and help with the new system. Another area might be treatment protocols or guidelines in one area that the team will be able to champion across the hospital. How these strengths can be used will become apparent as the work of putting a team into the field gets under way. A source of help in this area might be other specialist teams who are already established within the system. This will allow the identification of areas of shared interest and to understand their ways of working. An example is the acute pain team, whose path will inevitably cross that of outreach in day-to-day work.

DESIGN PROCESS

Once the scale and scope of the problems and deficiencies are understood then a careful assessment of the key design factors, combined with a clear understanding of the assets available, will lead to the 'best-fit' team design. Inevitably compromises will be made to produce the initial team but as the team develops it will be important to ensure consistently that any changes are in line with the original optimum design and are aimed at addressing priority areas. The factors that are important to consider when designing a team include:

1. team methodology;
2. team composition and size;
3. team organisation.

These are considered below.

TEAM METHODOLOGY

Critical care outreach teams can be broadly classified as either 'interventionist' or 'educationalist' (Table 2.1). However, in reality these are extremes of methodology with individual teams existing somewhere on a continuum between the two. An interventionist team directly influences patient care by taking an active, or even lead, role in the care of critically ill patients, whereas the educationalist team indirectly influences care by focusing on improving the knowledge base of the ward-based staff who would normally provide the care.

A team following the interventionist model will ask for referrals from the ward staff. They will then lead the care of the patient. The team may use a physiology-based scoring system, a list of referral triggers or a combination of both to identify patients to be referred.

A team whose approach is educationalist will focus on improving the overall care of the critically ill by training the staff caring for such patients. A small number of educators can affect the care of a much larger number of patients than they could personally care for, simply because of the 'gearing' effect of teaching a large number of providers of care.

Table 2.1 Comparison of outreach models

Interventionist	Educationalist
A critically ill patient will be directly managed by a team skilled in critical care	The ward staff are trained in the principles of critical care and can apply these principles to all patients preventing the deterioration of a number of patients
Will result in a small number of patients being managed to an extremely high standard	Will improve the care of a greater number of patients and educate ward staff to refer those requiring a higher level of input promptly
May tend to disenfranchise ward staff with potential for reducing benefits though likely to be welcomed once the patient is extremely ill	Educators may be perceived as lacking clinical credibility if they are never seen to manage a sick patient
The team is ideally placed to facilitate admission to ICU	There are already clear pathways by which patients are referred and admitted to ICU; these can be reinforced by an outreach team
Costly as the team will have to be large enough to provide 24 hour cover 365 days of the year	Gearing means that a small team will produce a greater degree of benefit; therefore it is relatively cheap

When faced with evidence of deficiencies in the care of critically ill patients, developing the service with an interventionist approach will initially appear attractive. This approach will mean that from the outset critically ill patients on the ward will be attended and managed directly by staff skilled in critical care, who are able to facilitate transfer readily to the ICU should the patient require it. However, there are a number of drawbacks that must be considered, not least of which is the cost of such an approach. Setting up a comprehensive new service to provide 24-hour cover for 365 days of the year including medical cover will be prohibitively expensive for most trusts. On the other hand setting up a service which is not 24-hour-365 creates issues of gaps in service provision and two-tier care. An interventionist service is limited as to the number of patients whose care it can influence and therefore will tend to concentrate its efforts on the extremely sick patient who is almost at the point of requiring an ICU bed. An interventionist team is unlikely to be able to turn these patients round without utilising an ICU bed and will therefore tend to become the route into critical care for most patients. The majority of critical care units already have clearly defined admission processes and inventing a new one does not seem to have any obvious benefits.

The relatively high cost of an interventionist team will mean that setting up a team with an educationalist approach will be attractive to fundholders simply because the team can be smaller and therefore cheaper than that required for an interventionist team. To some a single educator may be regarded as sufficient.

The team's methodology directly influences the responses of the ward-based staff and thus the efficacy of changes the team introduces. The interventionist approach may tend to disenfranchise ward staff by appearing to suggest that the ward staff are not capable of managing the patient, or that the team may be seen as interfering when they sweep in and start issuing orders and take over the care of patients previously cared for by the ward staff. Disenfranchised individuals tend to resist changes and may overtly or covertly delay referral, especially if they believe that intervention by the team is not required.

For an educational approach to effect any real change the team must be clinically credible, dynamic, effective educators and the changes that the team promote must be seen to improve patient care without significantly increasing the ward staff workload.

Clearly there are a range of approaches between the two extremes of educationalist and interventionist methodologies. I personally believe that the optimal approach for an outreach team is to be predominantly educational, actively supporting and guiding ward staff through the process of managing a critically ill patient and only intervening when required, but seeking to use any intervention as a tool for reinforcing the team's educational messages. Evidence to support assertions about which is the optimum model for outreach is eagerly awaited by the outreach community. While some significant improvements in outcomes were seen in initial evaluations of the medical emergency team (an interventionist model) (Buist et al. 2002), more recent evaluations from a randomised control trial did not support this model (Hillman 2005).

TEAM COMPOSITION AND SIZE

Deciding on the composition and size of the new outreach team is probably the most difficult step in the overall design process. A range of models exists, each model having its advantages and disadvantages, and so the model that is selected must enable the team to meet its objectives. These models include the following.

Solo educator service: a single individual responsible for organising and maintaining educational programmes and activity to support and develop ward staff. Clearly this team methodology has to be almost entirely educational. This model allows for little or no clinical input or 'team' intervention. This is the cheapest system to introduce; however, this model is likely to be the least effective way of improving care of the critically ill across a hospital. A single-handed educator will face huge problems simply generating the momentum to bring about major changes. This is especially true if there is any resistance to the desired changes. The service will close during holidays, study time and sick leave. But nevertheless there is the potential to improve care and the skills of ward teams.

Nurse-led team: a team of nurses possibly led by a nurse consultant. This type of team can be either educationalist or interventionist although the degree of intervention that a nurse-led team is able to make will vary significantly between hospitals, depending on the level of intervention and role expansion that the team members are comfortable with, as well as on the level of support from clinicians and managers. A team is more likely to be able to generate the momentum required to bring about change than the solo practitioner model. This is simply because a team can maintain a continuous level of activity throughout the year regardless of leave requirements. Single discipline teams may find it difficult to change the behaviour of other disciplines. However, the issues that that arise from consultant clinicians' reluctance to question colleagues' practice might be avoided by the assertive, credible and diplomatic nurse.

Multi-disciplinary team: a team of doctors, nurses and other allied professionals. This type of team can be either educationalist or interventionist. It is the most expensive option; however, this type of team is likely to be the most effective method of bringing about improvements in care. A team based on the multi-disciplinary model is uniquely placed to improve interdisciplinary communication and teamwork. It must be noted that the majority of teams publishing measurable benefits, and on whose work the recommendations included in the Department of Health's Document *Comprehensive Critical Care* were based, were all multi-disciplinary in nature (see for example Goldhill et al. 1999).

PERSONNEL INVOLVED IN CRITICAL CARE OUTREACH TEAMS

High quality care of the critically ill requires a multi-disciplinary approach. More specifically, it requires the knowledge base of a range of disciplines applied by individuals with appropriate experience of critical care.

The primary discipline of the majority of teams throughout Great Britain is nursing, with many teams consisting only of a single nurse. Nursing members of the team must have adequate clinical experience of critical care to be able to support emergency short-term critical care outside of an intensive care unit. One of the problems faced by many ICU nurses who move into outreach is that critical care is relatively straightforward within a well-equipped area such as an intensive care unit but can be extremely difficult to deliver in a side-room on a ward. This culture shock needs to be considered and allowed for with many teams organising attachments and/or development posts in outreach for ICU nurses. The learning needs of the outreach team are discussed more fully by Lee Cutler in Chapter 11.

The majority of doctors working on intensive care units in the United Kingdom are anaesthetists with smaller numbers of physicians and even smaller numbers of surgeons. A common problem faced by outreach teams is resistance from physicians and surgeons who believe they 'own' patients, and tend to refuse to allow input into 'their' patients' care. An experienced, diplomatic consultant practitioner actively involved in both the introduction and day-to-day activity of the team significantly reduces hostility from consultant surgeons and physicians, and thereby enhances team effectiveness. There is no point in 'drafting in' a reluctant intensivist as they are unlikely to be an asset and may well inhibit development if they are perceived as unenthusiastic about the new service.

Dieticians and speech therapists have a role to play in the team development and activity but do not necessarily have to be specifically employed as part of the team. The requirement for these disciplines to be included in the team will depend to a great extent on the activity and development of these disciplines within the hospital. A team based in a hospital with, for example, a well-developed acute physiotherapy service will gain little by employing their own physiotherapist; indeed the team will benefit to a greater degree by building both formal and informal links with the established service. However, it is interesting to read the case study by Alex Larkin regarding the more generic role of physiotherapists in critical care outreach.

There are clear advantages to having a range of disciplines involved in the development of the team. A simple way of developing formal links with an established service is to invite a senior representative of that service to participate in the outreach team planning meetings. Informal links are probably an outreach team's greatest asset; it is extremely useful to develop a number of reciprocal support arrangements with other specialist teams around the hospital and elsewhere. Simply ensuring that the outreach team carries copies of the guidelines and protocols of other teams – for example, the acute pain team – and adhering to those guidelines can reinforce informal links. Joint projects also serve to bring teams together, for example our patient group direction for commencing and titrating oxygen was developed and is used in collaboration with physiotherapy services, whereas our patient group direction for IV fluid bolus for the hypotensive patient was developed and used in collaboration with acute pain team nurses.

The initial size of the outreach team will depend on a number of factors, not least the funding available and the anticipated hours of cover required. Patients can become critically ill at any time and it would seem logical to provide a full time critical care outreach service, as has recently been recommended (DoH 2005; NCEPOD 2005). The hours of cover required will depend, to a great extent, on the team's chosen methodology. The level of readily available cover for patients should be be investigated before choosing the team's hours of cover. Out of hours is not always the problem one might expect. We were surprised to find that a simple audit of the time taken to get a doctor to attend an acutely ill patient revealed that there were greater delays in obtaining the attendance of a doctor, of at least a specialist registrar grade, during 'normal' working hours than out of hours. This was due to the conflict between daytime duties such as clinics, operating or endoscopy lists or consultant ward rounds and the provision of emergency cover.

If the team is to provide cover for less than the full 24 hours then a further problem arises in that to cover the maximum duration of time the staff should work individually rather than concurrently. However, members of the team need to meet to plan and organise the development process and at least have a handover period between shifts to maintain the service continuity. Some teams may choose to have an overlap period of a sufficient duration to allow a ward round of all outreach patients to occur on a daily basis. 'Grand rounds' undoubtedly have benefits for the team members in that they can discuss the patients' care amongst the team and arrive at a consensus before engaging with the ward staff. There is also the benefit that the round provides a regular visible presence of the team on the wards. There are, however, a number of potential problems with team ward rounds that must be considered; first is that outreach is about supporting ward staff to look after their patients and a round can easily become a task that detracts from patient care by occupying ward staff time; the second problem is that questions or problems may be left 'until the outreach ward round', resulting in further delay before a critically ill patient receives attention; the third problem is that ward staff are less likely to approach a large and confident group of staff to ask questions, and so educational opportunities will be lost.

The shift patterns and periods of cover varies significantly among outreach teams (Modernisation Agency 2003), with some nurses sticking to traditional early, late and night-shift patterns, while others work 'office' hours. Medical sessions for outreach will be less than nursing sessions and there will inevitably be times when a single practitioner is available for help and advice and others when several of the multi-disciplinary team are available (in larger outreach teams). It is a truism that nurses appear to seek support and advice from nurses and doctors from doctors. That being said, it is vital for the well-being of our target patients that the team leads by example and breaks down some of the barriers to effective care that result from interdisciplinary rivalries. Actively including medical staff in both formal and informal training of nurses, and probably more importantly doing the same for the outreach nurses in the education of junior doctors, will go some way towards engendering the mutual respect that is the basis of effective team working in acute critical situations.

Box 2.1 Case study

When the Doncaster Royal Infirmary outreach team was set up funding was obtained for two whole time equivalent F-grade nurses, seven anaesthetic consultant sessions, and consultant nurse input. During the initial set-up of the team and trialling of a scoring system on pilot wards it was felt that the team should cover as many hours as possible. The idea of a baton bleep passed between all members of the team allowed the greatest duration of cover. All calls were handled by the team member on duty when the call came in.

Initially there was some suspicion from the ward nurses when a consultant anaesthetist attended to show them how to read a central venous pressure manometer and from doctors when advised how to manage a critically ill patient by a nurse. The team was very conscious that it was breaking down barriers and the team members were careful to support their colleagues' opinions and specifically consult each other when possible in order to reinforce the message. The team continued with this policy for almost two years until they were able to secure funding for an increased number of nurses. The initial scepticism has been replaced by a high degree of trust in all members of the team and, more importantly, there appears to have been some improvement in interdisciplinary communication.

COMMUNICATION ISSUES

Clear, simple and effective communication strategies are essential in facilitating information exchange between the ward staff and the team, as well as within the team. There are a number of ways that this can be achieved. Some examples from practice are shared here.

First, as outreach is introduced, there is a need to publicise the team. All publicity is good and methods such as seminar presentations, newsletters, posters, business cards and pens with team details on work well in practice. Periodic advertising campaigns announcing each development, teaching session or team member change help to keep staff up-to-date. If the message is clear and relevant the hospital 'grapevine' will contribute to the dissemination of information.

It is essential that staff know when they can call the team. A few unsuccessful calls will soon put people off calling. If the service does not cover 24 hours consider advertising the hours of service on the wards by displaying posters, circulating rotas or even business cards with the hours clearly displayed. A single bleep number with a baton bleep passed between members of the team means that the staff do not have to refer to a list of numbers to find the right one. This should be supplemented by a dedicated phone number with an answer machine that is checked regularly.

Having a presence on the wards is important for a team who want to be consulted and who need to integrate with the multi-disciplinary staff throughout the hospital. If the team waits to be called then it may be ignored; wandering down to a ward if the team are not busy will publicise their presence. Relationships can be built and maintained with ward teams through link nurses in each ward area. These can be contacted on a regular basis and can attend link nurse meetings to enable feedback to the team as well as professional development.

Formal and informal links with other services play a vital role in clinical communication and coordination of care. 'Single point' contact for help reduces the workload for the ward staff and improves patient care. For example, the outreach team are asked to assist in the care of a patient with sputum retention due to pain from fractured ribs; the team advise on oxygen therapy and contact the pain team to manage pain relief and liaise with the on-call physiotherapy rather than telling the ward staff to contact the other two teams. Good communication and teamwork by the three services should mean that regardless of which team is called the others will be notified and the patient will benefit from coordinated multi-disciplinary care.

A team needs to give consistent non-contradictory advice. In order for this to happen the team members must effectively communicate between themselves. There is a range of ways that internal communication can be maintained including:

- maintaining separate notes within the patient's hospital files;
- formal team handover procedures or records;
- whiteboard or card systems with brief summaries;
- patient tracking IT systems.

The team communication system must not interfere with recording of actions or opinions in the patient's notes. Maintaining separate notes within the patient's hospital records will impair communication between the team and the ward staff, as the ward staff will be unlikely to note any advice. Writing advice or guidance within the relevant section of the patient's notes will at least have the benefit of being read by the ward staff, but it will be difficult to find for other members of the outreach team. A summary of the ward notes and a record of communications can be jotted onto a whiteboard or card-based communication system provided that these jottings are kept secure to prevent breaches of patient confidentiality. Whichever system is chosen it must be secure, effective and not replace the hospital record. We have found it convenient to leave a space for team communication on our audit forms. These are maintained in a folder carried by the outreach team member. Once a patient is discharged from outreach any jottings must be processed and destroyed.

AUDIT

Outreach is a relatively new service and as such it has to recognise that it will need to prove its worth. Audit is an important part of this process and should be built into the systems, processes and practices of the service. Creating a combined audit form and communication sheet is one example of directly linking activity to audit data. Single short focused audit projects assessing the proposed developments and therefore guiding the introduction process or the redesign process can be beneficial. Feeding the results of audits back to clinical staff is a very powerful way of initiating and evaluating change. Critical conversations around the findings of well-designed audit projects are about reality rather than opinions, assumptions, unfounded generalisations or dogma. Such a project is the topic of a case study that accompanies this chapter, while the evaluation of outreach is discussed by Paul Whiting and David Edbrooke in Chapter 13.

TEAM DEVELOPMENT

Clinical practice is continually developing and changing; a team fulfilling a single unchanging role is destined to become extinct. True 'Darwinian' evolution with random changes and natural selection would be impossible, and probably undesirable, to imitate. Instead a form of guided evolution should be used with the team introducing a number of potential solutions to specific problems and carefully auditing the effects of each solution to decide which solution is most appropriate for the area concerned. This approach will introduce changes in a way that involves the staff affected by the changes, in the process of system selection, thereby encouraging ownership of each change.

Below is a synopsis of some key developments in the process of establishing our outreach team.

CASE SUMMARY

Initial set-up

Having obtained the staffing for an outreach team a number of simple aims were defined. The team would follow the Department of Health's expert working groups guidance and attempt to avert ICU admissions, prevent the readmission of patients discharged from ICU and improve the care of the critically ill on the wards.

Understanding the problem

A review of the ward notes of ICU patients and observation charts identified a number of occasions where there had been a significant delay between a patient's observations deteriorating and the initiation of any specific supportive or resuscitative measures. It was unclear retrospectively why there had been such a delay.

Process mapping

A thorough assessment was made of the process by which a response is made to an abnormal set of observations. The hospital norm was for observations to be made by healthcare assistants using automated equipment. The observations had effectively been reduced to recording pulse, blood pressure and temperature although there were a number of wards that also recorded pulse oximetry saturations. Observations were recorded whether or not they were abnormal and the healthcare assistant moved on to the next patient. Some healthcare assistants learned to identify abnormal results but the hospital provided them with no formal training in interpretation.

There was then a delay in the process until a nurse or doctor reviewed the TPR chart. The nurses reviewed the TPR charts during the drug rounds and therefore this occurred a maximum of four times per day; the doctors reviewed the TPR charts during the daily business round though this was not guaranteed to occur every day.

Once the patient's deterioration had been identified there was potential for a further delay awaiting review by the medical team. This delay could occur for a number of reasons with the most common issue being the prioritisation of calls by the doctor. Doctors will prioritise calls based on a number of factors including the perceived urgency of the call, location of the patient and their own prior involvement in the patient concerned. It is not uncommon for a doctor to prioritise inappropriately a patient who is less sick but who has a nurse who is more effective at demanding the doctor's attention.

Once the junior doctor attended there was still potential for delays in initiating appropriate medical care, especially if this required calling in a more senior doctor, the 'If I call them in it will look like I can't cope' factor.

Following the process mapping exercise the key issues were defined as:

1. ensuring that every set of observations had a direct value to the patient;
2. developing a communication tool to allow the doctors to prioritise correctly;
3. providing some mechanism to encourage upward communication and senior involvement in the care of the most sick.

Selection of a scoring system

It was clear that a scoring system would need to be applied and the system chosen was that originally described by Morgan et al. This would allow a complete set of the standard ward observations to be scored and could be applied to all patients in that it did not require specialist equipment such as pulse oximetry or an expansion of the range of observations (as would happen if urine output was included). More complex systems were considered but it was felt that a simple and comprehensively applied system was preferable to a more complex system applied to a limited number of patients.

Introduction of a scoring system

The first phase of introducing the scoring system was the selection of the pilot wards. Asking for ward sisters to volunteer to be part of the pilot project went some way to ensuring that the first few wards had a degree of ownership in the project and were therefore likely to cooperate with its introduction.

The initial pilot was designed to answer two main questions:

1. *Who should calculate the scores?*
   There was a lot of discussion whether or not healthcare assistants would be able to correctly score the observations and, if not, whether the nurses would be willing to take over the observation rounds themselves. It seemed reasonable to develop a system of triggers that would tell the healthcare assistant when to inform the nurse and logically when the nurse should obtain a medical review.

   Every nurse and healthcare assistant on the pilot wards was individually taught and assessed in their understanding of the score and its associated communication protocol. It was readily established that not only were the healthcare assistants capable of scoring the observations accurately and rapidly but including this role in their duties increased the perceived value of the observations round in their minds and enhanced their job satisfaction.

2. *Should every set of observations be scored?*
   An audit comparing the scoring of every set of observations with the scoring of only those patients the nurses were concerned about clearly demonstrated significant delays in identifying the deteriorating patient if scoring only commenced once the staff were concerned about a patient. (This is presented as a case study which accompanies this chapter.)

Once the pilot phase was complete then the scoring system and an associated protocol for calling junior doctors was rolled out onto a small number of wards at a time allowing for intensive training of all staff and supervision of the introduction of the new regime. This staggered introduction has a number of benefits: it breaks the initial work into manageable sections, the teaching methods will become refined as the scheme proceeds so that the pace of introduction will steadily accelerate, mobile staff will move through areas covered by the team and word of the team's effectiveness will spread in advance of the introduction timetable. Probably the most important aspect is that developments can be tested on a small area currently under the spotlight, potentially avoiding a large-scale system failure.

As can be seen from the above synopsis, each step in the introduction process was heavily audited to ensure that the system was working in the way it was expected to. This robust evolutionary process remains in place with any newly identified problems and proposed changes being approached with the same approach within which the key stages are:

- assess
- consider alternatives
- trial and audit
- introduce.

PROCESS REDESIGN

In this final brief section I aim to discuss problems that the critical care out-reach team may face. These problems are not insurmountable but can be frustrating and challenging.

It can be extremely difficult to recognise problems with a service as an 'insider', especially when the service has been set up with the specific aim of identifying and correcting deficiencies in a system. There are a number of indicators that may help in recognising that all is not well. These can be classified as follows.

MINOR LACK OF COMPLIANCE WITH GUIDANCE

The ward-based staff do not seem to follow any of the guidelines or protocols produced by the team. There is clearly a spectrum of severity ranging from minor degrees of misunderstanding of the aim of the team's guidance through to a major refusal to involve the team. But indicators of problems will include: low uptake of the scoring system; low numbers of referrals to the team; low numbers of requests for aid; and poor attendance at teaching events.

MAJOR REFUSAL TO ACCEPT INVOLVEMENT OF THE TEAM

The doctors and the nurses specifically refuse to allow the outreach team to see patients; they may even conceal the level of sickness of a patient from the team because they believe that the team are interfering. They may refuse to apply the scoring system. In this situation there is a significant risk to patient care, especially if junior nurses and medical staff are confused about whose advice to follow.

Once the problem is detected the natural tendency of the team will to be to blame the ward staff for being unreceptive and to continue to try to explain to or teach the ward staff. This approach will reinforce the ward staff's impression that the team are being critical and result in further alienation. This worsening cycle needs to be broken before communication can be re-established and eventually trust redeveloped. It is essential to separate people from the problems and to depersonalise the situation. 'Seek first to under-stand . . . Then to be understood' (Covey 1989) is a simple summary of the steps to be undertaken. It is sensible to involve a respected independent person to try and investigate the issues that have led to the breakdown. Sepa-rating the people from the system will be a difficult but important step.

Asking everyone involved for their opinion and approaching people individually will take time, but is probably more effective than trying to arbitrate at
large and possibly heated meetings. Having listened to all concerned the
process of assessment of the true importance of the varying factors begins.
This may involve formally process mapping various aspects of the team's
proposed procedures and those currently in place.

Improving the quality of care a patient receives is rarely a contentious issue
and this is therefore often a good place to start the dialogue between team
and ward staff. It is important that the process remains focused on improvement and not correction of deficiencies. While the difference may be semantic
it is essential to establish a common purpose early in the discussions. The
critical question for the team to ask is: what are the implications for ward
staff of what we are suggesting? Staff may perceive an increased workload;
they may feel that there is a suggestion that they have been wrong, incompetent or ill intentioned in their practice or care. It could also be that staff feel
threatened, undermined and insecure. It is important to understand and
recognise these feelings and to point out the common ground – the patient.

Maintaining a dialogue between the team and the ward staff is essential as
the process has to remain a common project. Specifically looking at each
aspect of the management of a critically ill patient, mapping the journey and
looking at the patient's needs and the staff workload involved at each stage
can be a remarkably constructive process. It can be enlightening for staff from
a critical care background to work a shift with the ward staff, to see the problems associated with caring for a sick patient while maintaining the care of
the remaining patients.

The team's willingness to say 'perhaps we were wrong' and 'help us get this
right in the future' is sometimes difficult but humility goes a long way to
making personal links with individuals. It is probably the case that not all the
staff feel the same. Focusing on the willing and enthusiastic rather than the
negative and obstructive is a good strategy in the long term and it is surprising
how people change their opinions over time.

Critical care outreach is a process and not a solution and an outreach team
may have to accept that the process of change will be slower than they would
wish. The important thing is not to win all the battles but to win the war.

REFERENCES

Buist DM, Moore GE, Bernard SA, Waxman BP, Anderson JN, Nguyen TV (2002)
Effects of a medical emergency team on reduction of incidence of and mortality
from unexpected cardiac arrests in hospital: preliminary study. *British Medical
Journal* 324: 387–90.
Covey S (1989) *The Seven Habits of Highly Effective People.* New York: Simon &
Schuster.

Department of Health (2000) *Comprehensive Critical Care: A Review of Adult Critical Care Services.* London: Department of Health.

Department of Health (2005) *Beyond 'Comprehensive Critical Care': A Report by the Critical Care Stakeholder Forum.* London: Department of Health.

Goldacre M, Lambert T, Evans J, Turner G (2003) Preregistration house officers' views on whether their experience at medical school prepared them well for their jobs: national questionnaire survey. *British Medical Journal* 326(7397): 1011–12.

Goldhill DR, Worthington L, Mulcahy A, Tarling M, Sumner A (1999) The patient-at-risk team: identifying and managing seriously ill ward patients. *Anaesthesia* 54: 853–60.

Hillman K (2005) Introduction of the medical emergency team (MET) system: a cluster randomised controlled trial. *Lancet* 365: 2091–7.

Lee A, Bishop G, Hillman KM, Daffurn K (1995) The medical emergency team. *Anaesthesia and Intensive Care* 23: 183–6.

Modernisation Agency (2003) *The National Outreach Report 2003: Progress in Developing Services.* London: Department of Health and Modernisation Agency.

NCEPOD (2005) *'An Acute Problem?': National Confidential Enquiry into Patient Outcomes and Death.* London: NCEPOD.

2 Audit case study: scoring all observations compared with scoring only on concern

DAVID WOOD

This case study is presented as an example of how audit can help with service development and evaluation. The findings may be seen as context specific and not generalisable; however, they raise interesting questions about the use of track and triggers systems within acute ward settings.

BACKGROUND

If asked, most ward-based staff will state that they are quite able to identify a critically ill patient and really do not require a scoring system to tell them whether or not the patient is sick. I suspect that it is true that most doctors and nurses are able to identify a critically ill patient when they assess them. However there is a drive to increase patient throughput by shortening duration of stay and increasing the numbers of beds per ward. This is often combined with a reduction in the number of trained nurses on duty and their being replaced with healthcare assistants. As wards become busier and patient to trained staff ratios increase, then trained clinical staff will have less time per patient to make an assessment. It is increasingly common for healthcare assistants to make and record the patients' observations without reference to a trained nurse. As a result there is the potential for a significant delay before the observations are reviewed by the nursing staff. In practice most patients' observation charts are reviewed daily by the medical team and as part of the drug round by the nursing team. Intuitively it makes sense to have every set of observations interpreted by the person making the observations, who then immediately undertakes any required corrective action.

A set of observations should have an immediate value to the patient on whom they were performed. This cannot happen if the act of making the observations is separated from the act of assessing them.

Critical Care Outreach. Edited by Lee Cutler and Wayne Robson.
Copyright 2006 by John Wiley & Sons Ltd.

The process of making observations recognises that abnormalities in patient physiology are indicative of the severity of illness; a number of scoring systems have been devised as a way of indicating the degree of deviation of a patient's physiology from normal. These scoring systems usually result in a single number with higher values indicating increasing abnormality.

It would be possible to make a set of observations that have an immediate value to the patient if the person making the observations proceeded to calculate a physiology-based scoring system score on the observations at the time they are performed and who then ensured that any worsening changes in the score are brought to the immediate attention of the ward nurse. The trained ward nurse would then be able to use their training and experience to make a more thorough clinical assessment of the patient. Relying on a scoring system in this way could reduce the time spent by trained staff looking at charts as the trained staff would be directed to any patient whose condition was measurably changing and could commit proportionally more time to assessing the needs of the deteriorating patients.

As part of the introduction of critical care outreach in Doncaster a physiology-based scoring system was evaluated on a number of pilot wards. The strategy for the introduction of critical care outreach was that every aspect of the development would be rigorously assessed with alternative processes being simultaneously evaluated. It was hoped that this evolutionary approach would result in a system that was optimised for the hospital it was evolving within.

All healthcare assistants and nurses on the pilot wards were individually trained in the application of a scoring system; the healthcare assistants' ability to take reliable observations and to apply the scoring system correctly as well as their ability to calculate the score were all formally assessed before the early warning score pilot commenced.

WHAT STANDARD WERE WE AUDITING AGAINST?

A feature of audit is that it involves a process of data collection in order to make a judgement of the characteristics of a service as compared with explicit standards.

In this case the standards we wanted to achieve were, first, that all patients who were 'at risk' of becoming critically ill would be identified as soon as possible. Secondly, that their physiological aberration (detected through clinical observations) would be reported to the appropriate healthcare professional and that appropriate and timely action would be taken. It was our assumption that, in the context of busy wards where observation had been delegated to healthcare assistants, scoring only on concern could not achieve this. Hence we wanted every set of observations on every patient to be scored.

WHAT WERE WE TRYING TO FIND OUT?

As with all outreach teams we wanted to make a difference. We wanted to design a service which addressed our own specific, local problems. In this audit we wanted to know if we had designed the best system in asking for all observations to be scored. Alternatively, would critical illness go unrecognised or would the recognition be delayed if it was usual practice to score only on concern?

HOW WAS THE AUDIT SET UP?

Staff on one of the general surgical wards were reluctant to score all patients, but they were open-minded and willing to participate in audit and to change their practice if it could be shown that scoring all patients was best practice. The healthcare assistants on the ward were instructed to calculate a score only on observations of patients identified by the registered nurses as being 'at risk' or causing 'concern'. The healthcare assistants on the other general surgical wards were instructed to calculate a score on every set of observations performed and if the score was not zero (i.e. all physiological measures within the normal range) then to interrupt the observations round and inform the nurse in charge.

Reinforcement of the process and support of the ward staff were maintained for several weeks until the routines were well established and then data was collected over one month from observation charts.

HOW WAS DATA COLLECTED?

Data was collected on patients whose charts recorded a significantly abnormal early warning score (i.e. a score that had been defined as requiring the rapid notification of medical staff). Data collection involved the outreach nurses visiting the ward on a daily basis, reviewing all the observation charts and calculating early warning scores for the observations prior to the score recorded because of concern. Retrospective scoring of observations could only occur if a complete set of values had been recorded. The actual delay in triggering a score could be identified as the difference in time between the recorded 'triggering' score and a retrospectively calculated 'triggering' score. The numbers and times of incomplete sets of observations were also collected to assess the potential period over which the patient may have been deteriorating without this being detected.

FINDINGS

There was a clear difference in the thoroughness and completeness of taking and recording observations between the two approaches. In approximately 17% of patients, scored only on concern, the set of observations were incomplete. On the wards where all sets of patient observations were scored the observations were 100% complete. The process of calculating a score encourages the observer to make a comprehensive set of observations in two ways. First, it is impossible to complete the calculation without making a complete set of observations so the score effectively acts as a prompt sheet. Secondly, the process of calculating a score reminds the observer that the observations are part of a process and not simply a task to be completed. Interestingly many healthcare assistants reported that they felt that calculating and acting on a score improved their self-esteem by making them feel that the observations round was a worthwhile and important aspect of patient care.

In addition to those patients where the observations were inadequate there was objective evidence of patients in whom a deterioration, that would have produced a response if scored, had been missed. This delay in recognising the deterioration in physiology could be significant with one patient's observation chart indicating a change in the patient's condition that scoring would have identified over 72 hours before the staff noticed that the patient was deteriorating. In most patients identification of their deterioration was delayed by at least eight hours.

Overall there was a measurable delay or potential for a deterioration to be missed in 34% of patients who were scored only on concern when compared with scoring of every set of observations (Figure C2.1).

This audit made no attempt to standardise the frequency of observations and it is apparent that scoring the observations will only benefit the patients who have their observations made at an appropriate frequency. Daily observations could result in almost 24 hours of unrecognised deterioration.

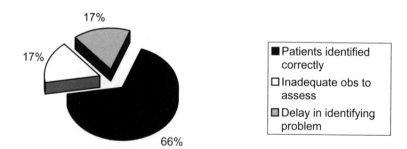

Figure C2.1 Findings from the audit of using the early warning score only on concern.

As a result of this audit it is hospital policy that every set of observations has a score calculated and all patients in whom the score is not zero are identified to the nurse in charge.

REFLECTIONS ON THE AUDIT AS PART OF SERVICE DEVELOPMENT AND EVALUATION

This audit demonstrates several simple but important principles. First, that setting standards is a useful starting point for developing a service. Secondly, changing practice can be challenging; however, professionals are usually willing to change practice given sufficient evidence that the change will result in an improvement. Lastly, working in partnership with ward teams to test your ideas of how things will work best allows learning to take place. This principle is key. It is not about being right: what really matters is that lessons are learned and this learning results in changes that improve care for patients.

II Clinical Practice in Critical Care Outreach

3 The initial assessment and care of the 'at risk patient'

JEREMY GROVES, JAYNE TAGUE AND LEE CUTLER

INTRODUCTION

Assessment and management of the 'at risk patient' is a primary role of the outreach team. This chapter provides an introductory level discussion that highlights and briefly examines some common features of initial assessment and abnormalities seen in patients at risk of critical illness. The discussion is aimed at the nurse or allied health professional who is new to outreach with the goal of orientating them to the focus of clinical work in this speciality. This is important since it differs substantially from the focus, culture and environment of intensive care, for example. It necessarily concentrates on basic and non-invasive assessment and monitoring. It involves supporting acute ward staff with the 'primary survey' of the at risk patient using an 'ABCDE' approach, recording of basic observations and use of 'track and trigger' scores, as well as initial intervention, priority setting and decision-making. These are themes within the chapter and are discussed with reference to literature as well as in the context of our own clinical wisdom which has been accrued over recent years working in critical care outreach. We have purposely attempted to be light on literature, and its critique, and instead focus on clarifying examples and on the common things we see in practice. In this way there is an economy of learning for the newcomer to outreach.

For greater depth of understanding of the physiology the reader is referred to key texts on critical care. For more advanced understanding of the principles of physical assessment the reader is referred to texts which deal with this area of practice. Finally, with regard to the evidence-based management of specific clinical problems the reader is referred to the contemporary literature as well as to Chapter 4 in this book which presents a summary of some of the common features of more specific assessment and management of the clinical problems that the newcomer to outreach will see in their everyday practice.

PREVENTION IS BETTER THAN CURE

'Prevention is better than cure': we are all aware of the sense in this statement but, in the context of critical illness, putting it into practice often presents a considerable challenge. The culture we are attempting to address through outreach services is a reactive rather than proactive one, which has developed over many years. In the hospital there are many obstacles that make clinical deterioration in a patient difficult to detect and prevent. The priorities of management in the contemporary NHS are target driven. Often these relate to time to 'be seen' rather than time for effective treatment.

Our wards are often under-resourced and the staff are pressured by an increased throughput of patients which places a significant administrative workload on clinical staff. Experienced nurses are often diverted from the ward bedside to non-clinical activities. Junior medical staff are often inexperienced. A period of rich clinical experience as well as appropriate support is required before they can realistically do the job they are expected to do as they first hit the wards – that of being the eyes and ears of their seniors and therefore troubleshooting. Junior medical staff may also be 'cross covering' patients from another firm in a different speciality with which they are unfamiliar.

In this context the wisdom of a simple and universally applicable approach to patient assessment and decision-making is invaluable. Such an approach is considered below, following discussion of 'early warning scoring' or 'track and trigger systems' (Modernisation Agency 2003).

ASSESSMENT OF THE ILL PATIENT IN A WARD ENVIRONMENT

If a patient is seriously ill it is often obvious to an experienced healthcare professional standing at the end of the bed with enough time and experience to look at the patient and think critically about their appearance. However, time, experience and critical thinking are not in abundance in the context of the busy acute ward environment.

Many times we have arrived on a ward to see a patient slumped in bed, their skin pale and sweaty, their head lolling forward, their eyes almost certainly closed, their cognitive state one of being oblivious to their surroundings and their breathing laboured or depressed. The attendance of the cardiac arrest team would have been not too far in the future.

This may be an exaggerated view but it does make the point that when people are very ill it does not require advanced knowledge to determine the fact. Sometimes when patients are admitted to the intensive care unit, the relatives may be angry, not because of their loved ones' illness, but because of the lack of recognition of illness or inaction in the face of it. Even they knew that something was wrong. How can we objectively detect the slide into critical illness at an early stage?

To answer this we have to consider what makes people ill. Simple you may say: bacteria, trauma and cancer, to name but three causes. This of course is true. However, we have many resident bacteria or abnormal cells in our bodies yet we do not become ill. William Osler, Emeritus Professor of Medicine at Oxford at the turn of the twentieth century, is quoted as saying that 'people do not die of their disease, but of the physiological consequences of their disease'. It is to the body's physiology that we turn to find the subtle signs that a pathological process is under way. The classic way of determining this at the bedside is through the use of basic observations.

OBSERVATIONS

The management of critically ill patients within a ward environment can sometimes be complex and a patient's condition can deteriorate quickly with little or no hope of recovery. Identification of seriously ill patients may be undertaken by clinical assessment of life-threatening signs of dysfunction of the airway, breathing or circulation. However, these premonitory signs may often be missed, misinterpreted or mismanaged by clinicians of all grades. This undoubtedly contributes to the morbidity and mortality of the patient, along with the economic consequences of dealing with them. McQuillan et al. (1998) found that up to 41% of admissions to their intensive care unit (ICU) were potentially avoidable, and sub-optimal care contributed to the morbidity and mortality in most cases. The early identification of such patients and the provision of a more timely intervention may help to prevent further deterioration of their condition and offer these patients a better chance of survival. Basic observations are a window into the physiological health of the body. Using them we can frequently map a patient's slide from physiological balance to the physiological derangement found in the critically ill. To ensure the best possible outcome we need to detect this slide as early as possible and to that end early warning scores (track and trigger systems) have been developed.

WHAT IS A 'TRACK AND TRIGGER' SYSTEM?

Track and trigger systems involve a monitoring tool that awards points for physiological values such as heart rate, respiratory rate and blood pressure when they are outside the normal range. The points awarded usually increase in value as physiological parameters worsen. Normal physiological parameters usually score zero. A total score is calculated and if this value is above a certain number then the patient has 'triggered'. The scores are quite crude and are not in themselves an indicator of organ or system failure or degree of dysfunction – rather that further assessment and intervention is indicated.

The implementation of a track and trigger system within the general wards provides the nursing staff with an objective measure with which they can make an assessment of the patient utilising the patient's routine observations. Many of the track and triggers systems are based on the modified early warning score (MEWS) developed at Queen's Hospital, Burton on Trent. MEWS was adapted from the early warning score developed by Morgan et al. (1997). These scoring systems were developed in response to studies showing that patients who had suffered an in-hospital cardiac arrest often had abnormal physiological values charted in the preceding hours (Wood and Smith 1999). Prior to the advent of the track and trigger systems, identifying patients who were ill relied upon personal experience and subjective judgement. Early warning scores are a more objective measure of the severity of the patients' illness, and empower individuals to seek assistance from a more senior member of the team.

The majority of hospitals have introduced some form of track and trigger system; however, it is acknowledged that these are not ubiquitous (NCEPOD 2005). Furthermore, even where they have been introduced, 100% compliance is a target for the future rather than a reality of the present (NCEPOD 2005). There is also considerable variation in the way the score is used in practice. Some hospitals employ a system where only selected patients are scored. These patients are those causing the nurse or doctor concern. Other hospitals have adopted a blanket approach whereby every set of observations recorded on the wards has to have an early warning score calculated. Evidence exists that scoring only on concern is associated with failure to identify at risk patients. Data to support this is provided in the case study presented by David Wood which accompanies Chapter 2.

The most common parameters seen include: conscious level, respiratory rate, heart rate, blood pressure, temperature and urine output. Some tools also include oxygen saturations. In addition to a simple scoring system, some outreach services have incorporated algorithms that guide the ward team in what to do in the event of a trigger or concern. This should primarily focus on the frequency that observations are recorded as well as calling for medical help to assess the patient. It may also involve calling or informing the outreach team of the 'trigger'. However, in order to ensure that ward staff and clinical teams are encouraged to maintain ownership of the problems calling outreach should not be the first response. Table 3.1 gives an example of the early warning score used in our hospital. Figure 3.1 gives an example of an algorithm used to guide staff in the event of a 'trigger' or concern (in our hospital we are currently scoring on concern).

DO TRACK AND TRIGGER SYSTEMS WORK?

Although track and trigger systems are now widely used in many hospitals in England, they have not yet been scientifically validated (Goldhill and McNarry

Table 3.1 An example of an early warning scoring system

	3	2	1	0	1	2	3
Conscious level		Newly confused or agitated		Alert	Responds to voice	Responds to pain	Unresponsive
Respiratory rate (breaths/min)	<8			8–20	21–30	31–35	>35
Heart rate (beats/min)	<40		40–50	51–100	101–110	111–130	>130
Systolic BP (mmHg)	<70	70–80	81–100	101–200		201–220	>220
Urine output (ml/h over 4 hours)		≤11	12–29	≥30			
Temperature (°C)	<34	34–35	35.1–36	36.1–37.9	38–38.5	38.6–40	>40

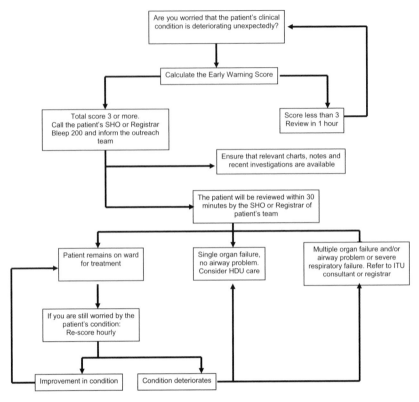

Figure 3.1 Example of an algorithm used to guide staff in the event of a 'trigger' or concern.

2004). There are however many studies showing that patients admitted to ICU or who suffer a cardiac arrest have abnormal physiological parameters in the hours or even days that precede (McQuillan et al. 1998; Kause et al. 2004; NCEPOD 2005). This suggests that many of these incidents may have been preventable if the abnormal physiology had been recognised earlier and acted upon. Abnormal early warning scores appear to be related to mortality. Goldhill et al. (2005) showed that as the number of physiological abnormalities increases so too does mortality, rising from a mortality of 4% with no physiological abnormalities to 51.9% with five or more. Stenhouse et al. (2000) carried out a nine-month prospective evaluation of a MEWS and reported that patients admitted to intensive care from surgical wards who had been put onto the MEWS scoring had lower admission APACHE II scores than those patients admitted from the surgical wards who had not been put onto MEWS, 16.6 compared with 23.5. Stenhouse et al. (2000) concluded that the MEWS appeared to lead to earlier referral to ICU. These findings and those that are growing within the wider literature resonate with our own experience and opinion regarding the usefulness of track and triggers systems. They are an essential clinical tool in the surveillance of hospitalised patients.

In summary, track and trigger systems are the safety net for patients in ward areas. They are what will alert the outreach team to patients who are deteriorating and who require more detailed, expert and intensive assessment and intervention. The next section gives a general and elementary guide to the process of assessing and intervening with seriously ill patients.

AN APPROACH TO THE SERIOUSLY ILL

This section might be alternatively entitled 'What to do when you are called to see a patient'. The feeling of anxiety that may be felt by novices, and even by more experienced practitioners, when they are called to see a patient is not uncommon. Having a simple and practical approach (perhaps photocopied and stuck to the inside of your outreach file) can be useful. When others are losing their head you will still maintain an air of calm confidence (at least on the outside!) as you ask fundamental questions in the process of assessing and facilitating timely and appropriate intervention.

We have summarised a practical approach to the seriously ill in Figure 3.2. This algorithm was developed by Lee Cutler and Judith Cutler for the 'RAMSI course' which is discussed in the case study that accompanies Chapter 5.

THE PRIMARY SURVEY

As you arrive at the patient's bedside ask for a clinical brief about the patient:

- name
- age
- reason the patient is in hospital
- what has happened for the staff to call you.

Then regardless of what assessment has already been undertaken, it is advisable to undertake a primary survey. The aim of this is to identify and immediately attend to any serious problems. Someone may have missed something or things may have deteriorated in the time since they last assessed the patient. In situations where cardiac and/or respiratory arrest is imminent assessment may take seconds. In situations where the patient's condition is serious but arrest is not immediately likely it is reasonable to take more time assessing more aspects of each system – but even in these circumstances the

---

Primary survey
A-B-C-D-E
Manage each problem immediately
Establish monitoring
Call for help

Secondary survey
History (from patient, charts and staff)
Full clinical examination
Investigations (review and request)
Call for help

Making clinical judgements and planning care
Do you know what the primary *problem* is?
Does the patient need further *investigations*?
Does the patient need *expert* review or *advanced intervention*?
Can the patient be managed in their current *location*?
Is this a *terminal* condition or event?

Definitive care and documentation
Document events and plan and communicate to all
Initiate referrals and facilitate definitive management

Figure 3.2 An approach to the seriously ill.

primary survey assessment should be structured and rapid. The assessment findings should lead to a rapid clinical grasp of the physiological problems even if the underlying diagnosis is uncertain. Problems with the airway should be addressed before breathing is formally assessed. This may mean delegating airway maintenance to someone while you progress to assess breathing. Problems with breathing should be formally addressed before circulation is assessed, and so on. This again may mean delegating – *'Please start oxygen by non-rebreathing mask and measure oxygen saturations.'* By the time you have assessed ABCDE you will have a lot to say to whoever you call for help or to review the patient, and you will sound credible.

- **Airway**   The key question you should ask yourself: *'Is the upper airway patent?'*

  Look for chest movement and work of breathing. Listen for the presence or absence of airway noises. Remember that any abnormal noises mean the airway is partially compromised. Feel for air on your cheek if breathing is difficult to detect. Employ appropriate airway maintenance manoeuvres or use adjuncts. These might include head tilt, chin lift or jaw thrust, insertion of oropharyngeal or nasopharyngeal airways or suction of the mouth and pharynx. In the unconscious patient side-lying, the recovery position may be safest.

- **Breathing**   The key questions you should ask yourself: *'Is gas exchange adequate?'* and *'How hard is the patient working to breathe?'*

  Look for signs of hypoxia pallor (an early sign) and cyanosis around the lips. Agitation and confusion or reduced consciousness may also be signs. Get someone to measure oxygen saturations and commence oxygen while you carry on assessing. How does the breathing look? Very rapid, very slow or shallow? Is there good chest movement? Is it symmetrical? Are accessory muscles being used? Feel the chest – it will help assessing chest movement and symmetry. Feel for tactile fremitus – the rumbling vibrations below your hands at lung apices and upper sternal borders that mean fluid/secretions in large airways. Listen to the chest. Are there breath sounds in all areas? Are there any added or abnormal sounds – wheeze, rhonchi, crackles, displaced bronchial sounds? (If you are unable to identify these sounds, get someone to teach you. It is not complex or difficult and is a very valuable clinical assessment skill.)

Key immediate respiratory interventions are as follows.

- ○ Clear the airway.
- ○ Commence and titrate oxygen – aim for SpO_2 of >95% (in chronic obstructive pulmonary disease (COPD) aim for 90–93%) (for more detailed guidance see Chapter 4).
- ○ Position the patient for optimum breathing; if conscious sit them up.
- ○ Relive bronchospasm.

- ○ Clear pulmonary secretions.
- ○ Manually ventilate with a bag-valve-mask if apnoeic.

- **Circulation**   The key question you should ask yourself: '*Is perfusion adequate?*'
   Have someone do a set of observations including pulse, blood pressure and temperature while you go to the patient. Feel their radial pulse for volume and rate. Feel the patient's skin at the peripheries and centrally and check their capillary refill time. Note that flushed extremities with a rapid capillary refill may be a sign of early 'hot' sepsis, and does not necessarily mean that perfusion is adequate. Tachycardia and hypotension, if an arrhythmia or acute heart failure has been excluded, may indicate hypovolaemia and the need for rapid IV fluid boluses. See Chapter 4 for more detailed guidance. Look at the urine of a catheterised patient for colour and volume, and request that it be measured hourly if you suspect circulatory and or renal dysfunction. Even if there is no one present to prescribe a fluid bolus, tell the staff to get some out in anticipation. Check to see if the patient has adequate, patent IV access. If not tell the staff to get a cannula out; delegate it to those present if they are able, or hang on until you've completed the primary survey before you set to work looking for a vein yourself.
- **Disability**   (or neurological deficit) The key question you should ask yourself: '*Is consciousness or mentation acutely altered?*'
   Ask someone to do a capillary blood glucose. Check the patient's responsiveness on the AVPU scale – are they Alert, do they respond to Voice, do they only respond to Pain (a good hard sternal rub or trapezius pinch), or are they Unresponsive? Check their pupils and ask if they have had any opiates or sedatives recently. This will establish the level of consciousness and identify the commonest causes. If they are unresponsive, go back and double check their airway and delegate its continuous monitoring to someone. If the BM is low get out some glucagon and 50% dextrose or whatever strength the ward has got. If you suspect benzodiazepine or opiate overdose, get out some flumazenil or naloxone respectively in anticipation.
   At this point assess for pain: ask the patient or palpate the abdomen of a surgical patient, especially if they are agitated or acutely confused – pain may manifest in this way.
- **Exposure**   The key question you should ask yourself is: '*Are there any obvious abnormalities or clues that will help direct interventions or further assessment?*'
   Expose the patient's abdomen and legs. Look at them for swelling (acute intra-abdominal pathology or DVT). Look at sites of intravascular devices for redness and possible causes of sepsis. Look for rashes and swelling anywhere on the body. Look at drains, wounds and stomas for obvious signs of large fluid or blood losses. Scan the body from head to toe for any other

abnormalities that may be a clue to acute deterioration, including behaviour and posture, e.g. rigors and twitching.

By now you will know a lot about the patient if only that you have ruled out lots of possible problems. If you have not done so already, get the staff to establish some kind of monitoring appropriate to the patient's condition and the situation you find yourself in. This might be 15 minute observations including HR, BP, RR, temperature, oxygen saturations, urine output and CVP or if you find yourself on a corridor with no equipment and only a student nurse. *'Keep your finger on a pulse and an eye on breathing. Shout if either stops.'*

Get some help if your survey reveals areas of concern. Bleep the most appropriate doctor – don't just start with the house officer and work up. If in doubt, go over the primary survey again. It is good practice to verbalise what you have found, what you are thinking and what questions are still unanswered. This allows others to know what you are thinking, avoids fixation, allows others to contribute and allows new ideas to be generated.

THE SECONDARY SURVEY

The next phase of the approach is to undertake a secondary survey. This is essentially a more in-depth and extensive review performed after initial resuscitative interventions have been initiated. However, while the phase of primary survey and secondary survey are described separately here, it is important not to think of them as completely separate. The primary survey should inform the secondary survey. It could be that as a novice in outreach you would generally call on a more expert or senior healthcare professional to undertake this. However, role expansion, advanced clinical skill development and appropriate and supportive policies for requesting investigations mean this phase is not beyond the nurse so long as consultation and communication with senior medical staff occur. The key point is: it doesn't really matter who undertakes this as long as someone does in a patient who is causing concern at primary survey where significant problems have been identified.

This phase involves a more comprehensive clinical examination, taking a more comprehensive history, requesting and review of investigations and consultation with others and/or calling for appropriate help.

It is usually the case that having undertaken a primary survey a reasonable grasp of the problems has been achieved, even if a definitive diagnosis or explanation remains elusive at this point. The implications for secondary survey are that the clinical examination, while necessarily more in-depth, can be more focussed and directed. For example, if the primary problem is clearly a respiratory problem the respiratory system can be thoroughly examined and investigated. It is important to talk over with the patient why you are there, what you are concerned about and for you to gain a general picture of their chronic and acute health problems and medical care including medicines and operations. It is possible to undertake a physical examination and take a history, as described here, almost simultaneously. A conversational style will help put the patient at ease and allow them to ask you questions.

It is useful then to withdraw from the bedside, find somewhere to sit and go over your findings as well as read the case notes and check any blood results or reports from recent investigations. This may usefully be undertaken as a group activity, especially if the right professionals are present, for example a senior doctor from the parent team and any other relevant staff. This is the phase of making clinical judgements and planning care.

MAKING CLINICAL JUDGEMENTS AND PLANNING CARE

Having undertaken a primary and secondary survey and consultation with the patient and relevant healthcare team members there should be a significant collective knowledge about the current health problems and their history and context. The series of questions presented here are aimed at guiding the process of making judgements and planning care.

Do you know what the primary problem is?

It is not unusual for patients to be taken to intensive care without a definitive diagnosis. However, after the kind of assessment described above, a grasp of the physiological problems should have been achieved, together with a more focused list of the differential diagnoses that one might have postulated at first sight of the patient. Knowing the most likely diagnosis, even though one might not have fully excluded others, is useful in directing care. This is especially the case in contemporary health care when 'care bundles' and evidence-based protocols are available to direct immediate and ongoing management. This question is key since it informs the other questions asked below as well as what information might be shared with the patient, family and other healthcare professionals at this point in the process.

Does the patient need further investigations?

If you have not been able to answer the question above conclusively then further investigation may well be indicated. Also if the severity of the condition has not been fully established it may be necessary to undertake further investigations. It may be appropriate that these are undertaken immediately or further resuscitation or admission to intensive care, for example, may be the priority with further investigations being undertaken a little later. Nevertheless their necessity should be added to the plan of care and the implications of any results considered and discussed with the patient and family – particularly if consent is needed.

Does the patient need expert review or advanced intervention?

In the case of a patient who is critically ill, expert review is essential. This means a senior critical care clinician as well as the patient's own consultant, or someone who has been in telephone contact with them should they be unable to attend. If the problem is a medical problem in a surgical patient, for example, then review and advice from an appropriate senior physician is required. Facilitating the timely involvement of the appropriate expert should be a priority.

Advanced intervention may mean organ/system support in the intensive care unit or emergency surgery, for example. Once a decision has been made and appropriate consent sought, facilitating and coordinating the necessary intervention should be a priority. However, ensuring that the patient is stable enough and adequately monitored and accompanied by appropriate medical and nursing staff for transfer is essential. All measures should be taken to ensure that any eventualities of moving the patient have been planned for.

Can the patient be managed in their current location?

This in part relates directly to the question above. If a patient requires advanced intervention they may well have to move clinical areas or even hospitals. However, this question also relates to patients where only moderate escalation of care has occurred. There are two relevant issues here. One is about what level of intervention can be safely managed in a ward environment, for example. This differs from ward to ward and from hospital to hospital, but the important thing is to check with the ward nurses. The second relates to the level of monitoring that is appropriate given the supportive interventions, the risks of deterioration, the underlying pathology and physiological aberration. For example, a labile blood pressure, fluid resuscitation, vasoactive drugs and the need for frequent blood sampling are all good reasons for having an arterial line inserted and moving a patient to a high dependency unit (if there's a spare bed!).

Is this a terminal condition or event?

The history, recently obtained or previously documented, the nature of the current problem, as well as the patient's response to resuscitative treatment so far will all be useful indicators of whether it is possible to treat the current problem successfully. It is not appropriate to consider the ethics of this issue at length here; however, it is appropriate to acknowledge the complexity of the issue of futility. What is important is that a decision is made and all the staff are well briefed about what that decision is. It is important, for example, to distinguish what care will be appropriate and when the decision will be reviewed, if at all. 'Do not resuscitate' decisions do not mean not to treat or resort only to 'TLC', and escalating treatment does not mean that *anything* will be done to preserve life. The parameters and context of any plan need to be explicit. This obviously has then to be communicated to all who need to know, including staff, family and patient, where appropriate.

DEFINITIVE CARE AND DOCUMENTATION

It is important that there is a clear, concise record of the process described here in the case notes. Finally any plan of care made needs to be put into action. This means that someone has to ask questions after each part of the plan is agreed upon: *'Who will ensure that that is done?'* and *'Who will review things later?'* Someone has to act with leadership in order to facilitate this whole process – as a member of the critical care outreach team that might be you!

SUMMARY

The complexities and inadequacies of modern health care within the acute ward setting place acutely ill patients 'at risk'. Deterioration in these patients may go unnoticed unless track and trigger systems are employed as a safety net directing team actions in response to basic clinical observations. However, for the outreach practitioner, who will be informed about patients who 'trigger', the wisdom of a simple and universally applicable approach to patient assessment and decision-making is invaluable.

REFERENCES

Goldhill DR, McNarry AF (2004) Physiological abnormalities in early warning scores are related to mortality in adult patients. *British Journal of Anaesthesia* 92(6): 882–4.

Goldhill DR, McNarry AF, Mandersloot G, McGinley A (2005) A physiologically based early warning score for ward patients: the association between score and outcome. *Anaesthesia* 60: 547–53.

Kause J, Smith G, Prytherch D et al. (2004) A comparison of antecedents to cardiac arrests, deaths and emergency intensive care admissions in Australia and New Zealand, and the United Kingdom – the ACADEMIA study. *Resuscitation* 62: 275–82.

McQuillan P, Pilkington S, Allan A (1998) Confidential inquiry into quality of care before admission to intensive care. *British Medical Journal* 316: 1853–8.

Modernisation Agency (2003) *The National Outreach Report 2003: Progress in Developing Services.* London: Department of Health and Modernisation Agency.

Morgan R, Williams F, Wright MM (1997) An early warning scoring system for detecting developing critical illness. *Clinical Intensive Care* 8(2): 100.

National Confidential Enquiry into Patient Outcome and Death (2005) *An Acute Problem?* London: NCEPOD.

Stenhouse C, Coates S, Tivey M et al. (2000) Prospective valuation of a modified early warning score to aid earlier detection of patients developing critical illness on a surgical ward. *British Journal of Anaesthesia* 84: 663.

Wood J, Smith A (1999) Active management should prevent cardiopulmonary arrest. *British Medical Journal* 318: 51–2.

4 Specific clinical problems

LEE CUTLER, ELAINE SHAW AND DAVID WOOD

INTRODUCTION

Acute outreach referrals commonly fall into four key categories: those of patients with respiratory problems, hypotension/shock, acute renal dysfunction and altered level of consciousness. The first part of this chapter is divided into four sections, each considering one of the key areas. The aim is to facilitate a broad, safe, approach to initial assessment and intervention. The latter part of each section then summarises important considerations for specific respiratory, cardiovascular, renal and neurological disorders. The second part of the chapter focuses on three other problems that may be commonly encountered by outreach practitioners and which often complicate critical illness, these are acute pain, delirium and inadequate nutrition.

The chapter is intended as a resource and includes algorithms currently used in practice and bibliographies on the conditions covered. It is not intended to replace in-depth specialist reviews, expert clinical knowledge or local protocols.

ACUTE RESPIRATORY FAILURE

Definition: where the respiratory system is unable to meet the metabolic demands of the body, resulting in reduced oxygenation ($PaO_2 < 8$ kPa breathing room air – type I respiratory failure) and/or retained carbon dioxide ($PaCO_2 > 6$ kPa – type II respiratory failure) (BTS 2002). These values assume no pre-existing lung disease. In patients with pre-existing lung disease a partially or uncompensated respiratory acidosis and/or $PaO_2 < 7$ kPa are more definitive.

Respiratory failure is a common life-threatening problem in the hospitalised patient. Some degree of respiratory dysfunction is a feature of many acute and chronic disorders which have the potential to result in respiratory failure. Early recognition of respiratory dysfunction can lead to prompt intervention and the possibility of preventing deterioration.

Critical Care Outreach. Edited by Lee Cutler and Wayne Robson.
Copyright 2006 by John Wiley & Sons Ltd.

There are some key broad principles that apply to the immediate assessment and management of acute respiratory problems where respiratory failure is suspected or evident.

However, there are also some dilemmas that outreach practitioners will face. Not least of these dilemmas is that of commencing and titrating oxygen because of the complex issues surrounding hypoxic respiratory drive in some patients with COPD. A rational approach to commencing and titrating oxygen for individual patients is required. Oxygen is probably the most commonly used but least prescribed drug in the acutely and critically ill. However, oxygen is only part of a complex set of issues that arise when assessing and intervening with patients who have acute, or acute on chronic, respiratory disorders. The key stages in the process should include:

- ensuring a patent airway;
- obtaining a brief history – ruling COPD in or out, considering if any chronic airflow limiting disease is asthma or COPD – in order to assess the risk of hypoxic drive;
- assessing for clinical features that indicate the need for oxygen to be commenced;
- commencing an appropriate amount of oxygen delivered by a fixed performance device and titrating the oxygen concentration to physiological targets;
- dealing with other immediate considerations (e.g. investigations, causes of acute deterioration, patient position);
- evaluation and ongoing collaborative management plan.

The algorithm presented in Figure 4.1 considers in detail these stages. The algorithm is the basis for a Patient Group Direction introduced so that non-medical outreach practitioners could commence and titrate oxygen. It is holistic and comprehensive enough to guide multi-disciplinary staff and ensure consistency of care. (Further discussion of the development and use of the algorithm is included in the case study by Elaine Shaw (page 133) on expanding the role of the nurse.)

SPECIFIC RESPIRATORY DISORDERS

ASTHMA

Clinical brief

Asthma can be defined as lung disease with the following characteristics:

- reversible airway obstruction;
- airway irritability secondary to an inflammatory response.

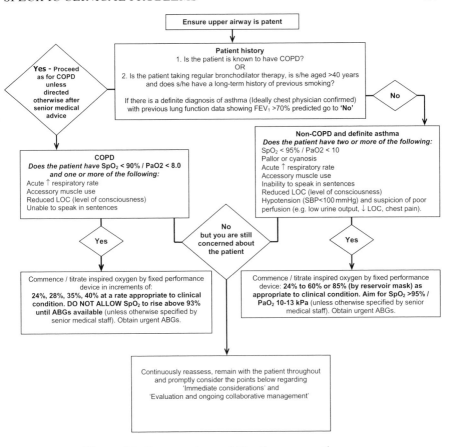

Figure 4.1 Commencing and titrating oxygen therapy.

Immediate considerations

• If not already done obtain urgent ABGs.
• If COPD believed probable (e.g. from history) obtain urgent ABG before administering >40% O_2.
• Request and review urgent chest X-ray if the patient has acute signs and symptoms of respiratory failure.
• Ensure that the patient is directly observed and that, as a minimum, temperature, pulse, BP, RR, SpO_2, LOC are recorded.
• Monitor the upper airway for compromise and intervene, or seek immediate expert help, to ensure the airway remains patent.
• Assess whether there is a need for secretion clearance from lower airways.
• Consider repositioning the patient for optimum breathing and gas exchange.
• Review medication (has necessary medication been omitted *or* has administered medication caused a 'reaction'?)
• Assess for extra-pulmonary causes contributing to the patient's current condition that can be treated (e.g. acute heart failure, pyrexia, pain, diaphragmatic splinting)?
• If the patient's condition is serious and does not improve after initial assessment and intervention, summon senior medical help immediately; remain with the patient and ensure that resuscitation equipment is to hand.

Evaluation and ongoing collaborative management considerations

• For COPD patients, if $PaCO_2$ is low give oxygen as for 'Non-COPD and definite asthma'.
• For COPD patients, if pH falls and/or $PaCO_2$ rises the patient may be receiving too much oxygen and a compromise target PaO_2 is needed. $PaO_2 \geq 6\,kPa$ is acceptable in the first instance for these patients but consider NIV if pH < 7.35.
• Consider whether intervention or advice from physiotherapy and/or anaesthetics/critical care is indicated.
• Consider if there is a need for CPAP/increase in CPAP (if F_iO_2 > 0.5 with refractory hypoxaemia and absence of hypercapnia).
• Continuous oxygen therapy/CPAP should be humidified.
• Consider if NIV is indicated (if $\uparrow PaCO_2$ & pH < 7.35 without acute severe hypoxaemia; also – cardiogenic pulmonary oedema unresponsive to CPAP).
• Consider the need for admission to critical care (HDU or ICU).
• Consider whether the patient needs mechanical ventilation ($\downarrow$LOC, exhaustion/acute asthma with $\uparrow PaCO_2$, impending respiratory arrest, refractory hypoxaemia despite $\uparrow F_iO_2$ and/or CPAP).
• Ensure all findings and interventions are documented, that senior medical staff are aware of the episode and that a collaborative plan of care is documented and communicated to the patient, family and multi-disciplinary team.
• Review resuscitation status and need to make explicit any limits on treatment escalation.

Clinical assessment

It is important to note that severity of attacks depends on two factors:

1. the degree of airway obstruction;
2. the ability of the patient to increase respiratory effort to compensate for the obstruction.

Hence a lesser degree of obstruction can still result in a life-threatening situation if the duration of the attack is sufficient to result in exhaustion.

Features of a severe attack

- cannot complete sentences in one breath
- use of accessory muscles
- respirations $\geq$25 breaths/min
- pulse >110 beats/min
- peak expiratory flow (PEF) $\leq$50% of predicted or best.

Features of a life-threatening attack

- silent chest, or feeble respiratory effort
- cyanosis
- bradycardia or hypotension
- exhaustion, confusion or coma
- PEF < 33% of predicted or best.

Diagnostic tests/investigations

- Peak expiratory flow less than 50% of predicted (or 50% of patient's normal PEFR) suggests a severe attack. Less than 33% commonly implies a rapid progression to a life-threatening situation.
- Arterial blood gases in the early phase of an asthma attack often show that $PaCO_2$ is low. A normal or elevated $PaCO_2$ is indicative of a severe attack. If a respiratory acidosis develops, the situation is life-threatening.
- Chest X-ray to exclude pneumothorax.

Key management considerations

If there are indicators that the situation is life-threatening then the patient requires the immediate attention of a critical care clinician for resuscitation and admission to intensive care.

The focus of management of severe attacks is to reverse the bronchospasm before the situation becomes life-threatening.

- Oxygen 40–60%.
- Salbutamol 5 mg (or terbutaline 10 mg) nebulisers driven by oxygen every 15 minutes until there are signs of improvement – when the frequency can be reduced.
- Ipratropium 0.5 mg 4–6 hourly by oxygen driven nebuliser.
- Steroids – either IV hydrocortisone 100 mg or prednisolone tablets 40–60 mg stat followed by regular oral prednisolone 40–60 mg daily if improving or IV hydrocortisone 100 mg 6 hourly if not.
- Aminophyline infusion with a bolus if the patient has had no previous Theophylline (BTS and SIGN 2004).
- IV fluid replacement as severe attacks mean that the patient has high evaporative losses and is usually too breathless to drink.
- An IV bolus of magnesium has been shown to be of benefit. Infusions of magnesium should only be used in a monitored environment because of the risks of adversely affecting muscle function.
- Consider the cause of the attack and treat with antibiotics if the cause does appear to be infective.
- If the patient appears to be becoming distressed then the situation is deteriorating and may well be becoming life-threatening. Do *not* give sedatives.
- Repeat arterial blood gases are helpful especially if the patient does not appear to be responding to treatment. (NB arterial punctures can be painful and distressing for the patient.) Good technique with use of local anaesthesia is essential.
- No sedatives of any kind.

CHRONIC OBSTRUCTIVE PULMONARY DISEASE (COPD)

Clinical brief

'COPD is characterised by airflow obstruction. The airflow obstruction is usually progressive, not fully reversible and does not change markedly over several months' (NICE 2004, p. 5). The disease is predominantly caused by smoking (NICE 2004). COPD refers to a group of disorders that include emphysema and chronic bronchitis. Emphysema involves destruction of alveoli and a tendency of small airways to collapse due to irreversible destruction of elastin. Chronic bronchitis is characterised by irritation, inflammation and oedema of airways and excess mucus production. While these are very different conditions, they often coexist in individuals with COPD (Celli et al. 1995).

A diagnosis of COPD should be made on the basis of history, physical examination and evidence of airflow obstruction from spirometry (FEV_1 < 80% predicted and FEV_1/FVC < 0.7).

'An exacerbation is a sustained worsening of the patient's symptoms from their usual stable state which is beyond normal day-to-day variations, and is acute in onset' (NICE 2004, p. 30). An exacerbation is usually associated with increased:

- breathlessness
- cough
- sputum purulence
- sputum volume.

Assessment and investigation in exacerbation – key points

- chest X-ray
- arterial blood gases
- ECG
- full blood count
- U&Es
- theophylline level (for those already receiving theophylline)
- sputum microscopy and culture if purulent
- blood culture (if pyrexial) (NICE 2004).

Key management considerations in acute exacerbation

- supplemental oxygen (target SaO_2 90–93%) and monitor blood gases for hypercapnia (NICE 2004)
- nebulised bronchodilators (salbutamol and ipratropium)
- antibiotics (if sputum more purulent than patient's normal) checked against laboratory culture and sensitivity when available
- oral prednisolone 30mg daily for 7–14 days or (IV hydrocortisone as an alternative if oral route inappropriate)
- IV theophylline only as an adjunct where there is inadequate response to inhaled bronchdilators
- respiratory physiotherapy to aid sputum clearance (NICE 2004)
- non-invasive ventilation ($\uparrow PaCO_2$ and pH < 7.35 without acute severe hypoxaemia)
- CPAP ($F_IO_2 > 0.5$, refractory hypoxaemia and absence of hypercapnia)
- plan of care covering what to do in the event of deterioration and what ceiling on therapy is appropriate, especially whether mechanical ventilation is deemed appropriate
- where appropriate, early referrals and admission to high dependency care/ intensive care units will minimise the sequelae of severe or protracted respiratory failure (BTS 2002).

Intravenous rehydration and enteral tube feeding in extreme dyspnoea are essential parts of good general care, and should not be forgotten.

PNEUMONIA

Clinical brief

Pneumonia can be defined as an acute infection of lung parenchyma including alveolar spaces and interstitial tissue; involvement may be confined to an entire lobe, a segment of a lobe, alveolar contiguous to bronchi, or interstitial tissue. These distinctions are generally based upon X-ray findings (Ruch 1999).

Assessment and investigation – key points

- chest radiograph
- blood cultures (preferably prior to commencement of antibiotic treatment)
- assessment of oxygenation (arterial blood gases and pulse oximetry)
- sputum culture and gram staining
- specific tests as advised locally by microbiologists especially if not improving (e.g. culture, serology, antigen tests and complement fixation tests)
- FBC
- U&E
- LFT
- CRP (BTS 2001).

Additional points from the history that may be useful in determining clinical management:

- history of travel abroad
- previous respiratory disease (and testing, e.g. spirometry)
- previous pulmonary infections
- immune status
- coexisting disease (e.g. diabetes, malignancy, HIV, cardiac disease, chronic neurological illness, renal disease) (Niederman 2001).

Adverse prognostic features

- age > 50 yrs
- presence of coexisting disease
- new mental confusion
- uraemia (>7 mmol/l)
- tachypnoea (RR > 30/min)
- hypotension (SBP < 90 mmHg and/or DBP < 60 mmHg)
- hypoxaemia (SpO_2 < 92%, PaO_2 < 8 kpa)
- bilateral or multilobe involvement (from chest radiograph) (BTS 2001).

Management considerations – key points

- oxygen therapy (humidified) and monitoring of oxygenation
- antibiotics (and microbiologist advice)
- analgesia for pleuritic pain if required
- chest physiotherapy
- hydration assessment and IV fluid hydration
- nutritional therapy/supplements
- rest
- antipyretics.

In those who are critically ill

- additional measures to maintain adequate oxygenation and ventilation (CPAP, NIV or mechanical ventilation)
- assistance with sputum clearance (e.g. 'Minitracheostomy')
- serial CRPs and chest radiographs (especially if not improving)
- therapeutic bronchoscopy
- early identification and management of sepsis (including IV fluid resuscitation, inotropes or vasoconstrictors and microbiologist involvement in antibiotic therapy).

ACUTE RESPIRATORY DISTRESS SYNDROME (ARDS) AND ACUTE LUNG INJURY (ALI)

Clinical brief

ARDS and ALI are part of a clinical syndrome of severe acute lung injury involving diffuse alveolar damage and non-cardiogenic pulmonary oedema. There are no pathognomonic tests for these but diagnostic criteria have been agreed internationally (Figure 4.2).

ARDS: - Acute onset of respiratory failure   - Diffuse bilateral infiltrates on frontal chest X-ray   - No clinical evidence of left atrial hypertension (PCWP < 18 mmHg)   - PaO_2/FiO_2 < 200 mmHg (26.6 kPa)   - ALI same as ARDS but PaO_2/FiO_2 < 300 mmHg (40 kPa)   (Bernard et al. 1994)

Figure 4.2 Diagnostic criteria for ARDS and ALI.

Assessment and investigations – key points

- CXR
- blood gases

- haemodynamic monitoring (CVP/PAP to exclude left atrial hypertention)
- thorough history and examination to identify possible aetiological factors (e.g. sepsis, pancreatitis, pneumonia, trauma, disseminated intravascular coagulation, extensive burns).

Management considerations – key points

- oxygen
- CPAP
- fluid management to prevent intravascular overload while maintaining adequate organ perfusion
- prompt referral to critical care consultant to facilitate early mechanical ventilation
- vigilance to prevent, identify and treat secondary/nosocomial infections
- nutrition (enteral if possible) to nourish and promote the normal gastro-intestinal mucosal barrier function.

CIRCULATORY SHOCK

Definition: 'The state in which profound and widespread reduction of effective tissue perfusion leads first to reversible and then, if prolonged, to irreversible cellular injury' (Kumar and Parrillo 2001, p. 373).

The three aetiological classifications of shock most commonly seen in outreach practice are septic, hypovolaemic, and cardiogenic shock. The final common pathway, that of multi-organ dysfunction syndrome (Kumar and Parrillo 2001), and the high associated mortality, demands that the prompt identification and management of shock be a high priority for outreach staff.

The outreach practitioner may be 'on scene' early in the disease process and may serve as valuable means of initial assessment, intervention and referral to specialist clinicians. Transfer to a unit for specialist care and monitoring may also be facilitated by the outreach practitioner and overall support, education and leadership is a further invaluable contribution that can be made.

The in-depth management of these three key shock states is not considered here. However some key points are offered. An approach to the shocked/hypotensive patient is presented below in a clinical algorithm (Figure 4.3) and key issues related to assessment and management are briefly reviewed. The algorithm is in current use in practice as a basis for intravenous fluid challenges by nursing staff acting under a Patient Group Direction.

The key stages in the process described by the algorithm are:

- assessment of airway and breathing and immediate measures to manage problems identified;
- assess the circulation for features of shock or impending shock because of recent/ongoing fluid losses;

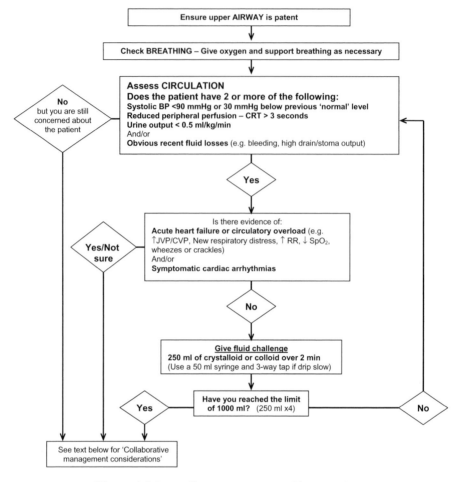

Figure 4.3 Immediate management of hypotension.

Collaborative management considerations

- Consider the need for urgent expert medical help (general concern for the patient, management of new and symptomatic cardiac arrhythmias, ongoing fluid resuscitation).
- Ensure that the patient is directly observed and that as a minimum temperature, pulse, BP, RR, SpO₂, LOC are recorded.
- Ensure adequate, patent IV access.
- Catheterise and record hourly urine output.
- Review full history and recent events.
- Review and request investigations as indicated (e.g. U&E, FBC, clotting, ECG, CXR).
- Examine the patient systematically in order to identify possible causes of the hypotension/deterioration.
- Is there evidence of sepsis? (temperature >38°C or <36°C, pulse >90, RR > 20 or PaCO₂ < 4.3 kPa, WBC > 12,000).
- Is there evidence of haemorrhage? (haematemesis, melaena, abdominal distension, falling Hb).
- Review medication (has necessary medication been omitted *or* has administered medication caused a 'reaction'?).
- Does the patient need continuous/invasive cardiovascular monitoring (and admission to a critical care unit)?
- Are inotropes or vasopressors indicated to treat hypotension refractory to fluid boluses?
- Ensure all findings and interventions are documented, that senior medical staff are aware of the episode and that a collaborative plan of care is documented and communicated to the patient, family and multi-disciplinary team.

- assess for evidence of heart failure/circulatory overload or symptomatic cardiac arrhythmias where bolus IV fluids would be contraindicated;
- give IV fluid challenges and reassess after each challenge to evaluate its effects and repeat if indicated up to a volume limit of 1000–1500ml;
- review thoroughly and formulate a plan to monitor and collaboratively manage the patient.

SPECIFIC CIRCULATORY DISORDERS

CARDIOGENIC SHOCK

Clinical brief

Cardiogenic shock is an emergency carrying a high mortality rate. It results from the failure of the heart as a pump, usually as a result of myocardial infarction. Elevated preload (CVP), reduced cardiac output and increased SVR (peripheral 'shutdown') are all key features. Congestive heart failure (volume overload) may present similarly though it is generally less serious in its effects on organ perfusion and is more easily managed through off-loading intravascular volume. Acute cardiac arrhythmias that cause haemodynamic compromise may also cause pump failure and mimic congestive heart failure.

Assessment and investigations – key points

- ABCDE approach including limited but directed history and examination
- 12 lead ECG and bedside rhythm monitoring
- chest X-ray
- echocardiography
- arterial blood gases (including lactate levels to evaluate the severity of reduced tissue perfusion)
- urea and electrolytes, Mg^{2+}, Ca^{2+}
- full blood count (Hb, WBC, platelets)
- frequent systemic arterial pressure monitoring (preferably continuous by arterial cannulation)
- urinary catheterisation and hourly urine output.

The haemodynamic criteria for the diagnosis of cardiogenic shock include: systolic BP < 90mmHg > 30min, cardiac index <2.2l/min/M^2 and pulmonary artery wedge pressure >15mmHg (Hollenburg and Parillo 2001). However, without the facilities to perform the latter of these two measurements outside the critical care unit, the practitioner may consider a seminal classification system for patients following myocardial infarction (Killip and Kimball 1967)

(Table 4.1). The subsets outlined differ somewhat physiologically from those defined with the advent of right heart catheterisation (Forrester et al. 1977) and, in the context of modern cardiology, their predictive value differs from that originally proposed (Madais 2000). However, as a 'blunt tool' for assessing severity in the presence of other non-invasive parameters they have some value in the outreach context (Connaughton 2001).

Management considerations – key points

- supplemental oxygen
- CPAP or NIV for refractory hypoxaemia
- venous access preferably – central venous access to evaluate preload
- analgesia (and anxiolysis).

After initially identifying cardiogenic shock or significant cardiac failure, referral to a cardiologist and specialist cardiac/coronary care unit is a high priority. Close and continuous monitoring of cardiac function and organ perfusion is key and strategies to optimise these need to be tailored to the individual patient and their physiology, they may include:

- diuretics or fluid challenges
- inotropes
- vasopressors or vasodilators
- reperfusion strategies (thrombolytic therapies, cardiac catheterisation, angioplasty, CABG) (Hollenburg et al. 1999).

Table 4.1 Clinical features of cardiac failure

Killip class	Clinical features of cardiac failure
I	No failure
II	Mild to moderate; S_3; crackles in <50% of lungs
III	Severe; S_3; crackles in >50% of lungs
IV	Cardiogenic shock

HYPOVOLAEMIC SHOCK

Clinical brief

Hypovolaemic shock is probably the most common form of shock that will be seen by critical care outreach practitioners and should be considered an emergency. It occurs as a result of inadequate fluid volume in the intravascular space Common causes are dehydration, haemorrhage, diarrhoea and/or vomiting, polyuria, third space losses with increased vascular permeability. However, vasodilation from a number of causes may also result in a relative hypovolaemic state (sepsis, spinal injury, drugs and toxins, anaphylaxis).

Assessment and investigations – key points

- ABCDE approach including limited but directed history, examination and review of charts to determine the cause of fluid losses/vasodilation
- rapid estimation of the degree of hypovolaemia (to this end Table 4.2 may serve as a useful guide)
- arterial blood gases (including lactate levels to evaluate the severity of reduced tissue perfusion – normal values are 0.3–1.3 mmol/l; values > 4 indicate shock)
- full blood count (Hb, WBC, platelets)
- clotting screen
- urea and electrolytes
- 12 lead ECG, especially if chest pain present or myocardial ischaemia suspected
- frequent systemic arterial pressure monitoring
- urinary catheterisation and hourly urine output
- central venous pressure trend monitoring
- assessment associated with confirming the aetiology where the cause of shock is unclear or may be multi-factorial (e.g. blood cultures, C-reactive protein – septic; troponin – cardiogenic; drug history, mast cell tryptase – anaphylactic).

Table 4.2 Classification of hypovolaemic shock (estimates based on a 70 kg person)

	Class 1	Class II	Class III	Class IV
Blood loss (% of blood)	<15%	15–30%	30–40%	>40%
Blood loss (ml)	<750	750–1500	1500–2000	>2000
Heart rate	<100	>100	>120	>140
SBP	Unchanged	Normal	↓	↓↓
DBP	Unchanged	↑	↓	↓↓
Pulse pressure	Normal	↓	↓	↓↓
Capillary refill	Normal	>2s	>2s	Undetectable
Respiratory rate	14–20	20–30	30–40	>35
Urine output	>30 ml/h	20–30	5–15	Negligible
CNS/mental status	Alert	Anxious	Anxious and confused	Confused and lethargic/ unconscious

Source: Reproduced with permission from American College of Surgeons' Committee on Trauma, Advanced Trauma Life Support for Doctors (ATLS) Faculty Manual, 1997; 6th Edition, Chicago: American College of Surgeons, 1997.

Management considerations – key points

- the goal is restoration of adequate circulating volume and organ perfusion
- rapid, multiple, wide bore cannulation (central venous access if/when possible)
- rapid administration of intravenous fluid – adjusted according to type and volume of losses (crystalloid/colloid, blood)
- fluid challenges in suspected hypovolaemia should be given at 500–1000 ml crystalloid or 300–500 ml colloid over 30 min and repeated based on response (Dellinger et al. 2004)
- supplemental oxygen therapy
- correction of electrolyte imbalances
- administration of blood products in coagulopathy/haemorrhage/large transfusion
- inotropes/vasopressors as adjuvant to fluid resuscitation.

When part of a sepsis-induced hypovolaemia and hypoperfusion 'early goal-directed therapy' has been shown to improve survival in patients presenting with septic shock (Rivers et al. 2001). Because hypovolaemia and sepsis often coexist this evidence should clearly influence practice. Rivers et al. (2001) used the following goals for the first six hours of resuscitation:

- CVP 8–12 mmHg
- mean arterial pressure ≥ 65 mmHg
- urine output ≥0.5 ml/kg/h
- mixed venous oxygen saturation ≥70% (central venous oxygen saturations are deemed equivalent (Dellinger et al. 2004)).

Failure to achieve mixed venous oxygen saturations of >70% should be managed by packed cell transfusion to achieve haematocrit >30% and/or dobutamine infusion up to 20 µg/kg/min (Rivers et al. 2001).

'SEPTIC SHOCK', 'SEVERE SEPSIS' AND 'SIRS'

Clinical brief

The generalised term 'sepsis' describes a systemic inflammatory response to infection which is progressive and injurious (Levy et al. 2003). A consensus on other, more specific descriptors such as 'septic shock' (presenting as hypotension and poor perfusion despite fluid resuscitation), 'severe sepsis' (sepsis with organ dysfunction) and 'SIRS' (the systemic inflammatory response to a variety of severe clinical insults – not just infection) has developed over recent years (ACCP/SCCM 1992; Levy et al. 2003). These syndromes are common in the hospitalised adult. Recognition and appropriate early intervention is crucial to improving outcome in patients with 'sepsis' (ACCP/ SCCM 1992; Rivers et al. 2001; Dellinger et al. 2004).

Recent detailed diagnostic criteria have been agreed internationally. These are thought to be useful in identifying 'most' patients with minimal sacrifice of specificity (Levy et al. 2003) (Figure 4.4).

Assessment and investigations – key points

- ABCDE approach including limited but directed history, examination and review of charts
- arterial blood gases (including lactate levels to evaluate the severity of reduced tissue perfusion)
- full blood count (Hb, WBC, platelets)

- Infection (documented or suspected)
- General variables:
  - o Fever or hypothermia (core temperature > 38.3 °C or < 36 °C)
  - o Tachycardia (> 90 or > 2 SD above normal value for age)
  - o Tachypnoea
  - o Altered mental status
  - o Significant oedema or positive fluid balance (> 20 ml/kg over 24 hours)
  - o Hyperglycaemia (> 7.7 mmol/l) in the absence of diabetes
- Inflammatory variables:
  - o Leukocytosis (WBC > 12,000 µl)
  - o Leukopenia (WBC < 4000 µl)
  - o Normal WBC with > 10% immature forms
  - o Plasma C-reactive protein > 2 SD above normal value
  - o Plasma procalcitonin > 2 SD above normal value
- Haemodynamic variables:
  - o Hypotension (< 90 mmHg, MAP <70 mmHg, or SBP decrease > 40 mmHg in adults or 2 SD below normal for age)
  - o SvO_2 > 70%
  - o Cardiac index > 3.5 l/min/m^2
- Organ dysfunction variables:
  - o Arterial hypoxaemia (PaO_2/FiO_2 < 300 mmHg)
  - o Acute oliguria (urine output < 0.5 ml/kg/h)
  - o Creatinine increase > 0.5 mg/dl
  - o Coagulation abnormalities (INR > 1.5 or APTT > 60 s)
  - o Ileus (absent bowel sounds)
  - o Thrombocytopenia platelet count < 100,000 µl)
  - o Hyperbilirubinaemia (plasma total bilirubin > 70 mmol/l)
- Tissue perfusion variables:
  - o Hyperlactataemia (> 1 mmol/l)
  - o Decreased capillary refill or mottling

Figure 4.4 Diagnostic criteria for septic shock, severe sepsis and SIRS.

- C-reactive protein
- clotting screen
- urea and electrolytes
- plasma glucose
- liver function tests
- 12 lead ECG (if arrhythmias or myocardial ischaemia suspected)
- chest X-ray (especially if chest infection is a possible cause of sepsis)
- frequent systemic arterial pressure monitoring
- temperature, pulse and respiratory rate monitoring
- urinary catheterisation and hourly urine output
- central venous pressure trend monitoring
- blood cultures prior to commencement of antibiotic therapy; at least two – one drawn percutaneously and one from each vascular access device if in situ >48h (Weinstein et al. 1983, cited in Dellinger et al. 2004)
- other cultures where relevant (e.g. urine, sputum, CSF, drain fluid, wound swabs).

Management considerations – key points

For patients with sepsis, in particular septic shock and severe sepsis, there may be two stages to the management strategy for the outreach team. Initial rapid assessment, resuscitation and transfer may characterise the first phase. Following this, critical care admission and ongoing monitoring and management may be more invasive and extensive. Some elements of the second phase might be commenced by the well-equipped 'interventionist' outreach team, or at least anticipated. However, each situation should be dealt with individually.

Initial management

Management of severe sepsis or septic shock should begin as soon as it is recognised. The goals of therapy are aimed at maximising tissue perfusion in the first six hours. The physiological targets should be:

- CVP 8–12 mmHg
- mean arterial pressure ≥65 mmHg
- urine output >0.5 ml/kg/h
- central venous (superior vena cava) or mixed venous oxygen saturations ≥70% (Rivers et al. 2001)

Treatments

- 'Early goal-directed therapy' (Rivers et al. 2001) aimed at achieving the above physiological targets, including fluid challenges (500–1000 ml crystalloid or 300–500 ml colloid over 30 min. Where mixed venous oxygen saturations are not ≥70% despite volume replacement to a CVP of 8–12 mmHg, transfuse packed red cells to a haematocrit of ≥30% and/or administer dobutamine infusion up to 20 μg/kg/min.

- Vasopressors +/− inotropes as adjuvant to fluid resuscitation in refractory hypotension (Dellinger et al. 2004).
- Intravenous antibiotic therapy should be commenced within the first hour of recognition of severe sepsis, after appropriate cultures have been obtained (Dellinger et al. 2004).
- 'Source control' – identification of infective focus and appropriate intervention (Jimenez and Marshall 2001, cited in Dellinger et al. 2004).
- Intravenous steroids (200–300 mg/day for 7 days) for patients with septic shock requiring vasopressor and having relative adrenal insufficiency (cortisol increase <9 μg/dl after ACTH) (Annane et al. 2002, cited in Dellinger et al. 2004).
- Recombinant Human Activated Protein C (rhAPC) should be commenced as soon as possible in those at high risk of death (APACHE II >25, septic shock, sepsis induced multiple organ failure or sepsis induced ARDS) in the absence of contraindications (Bernard et al. 2001, cited in Dellinger et al. 2004; Green et al. 2005).
- Platelet transfusion (if platelets between 5 and $30 \times 10^9/l$) in anticipation of the insertion of invasive lines or if surgery is planned (ASA, 1996 – cited in Dellinger et al. 2004).
- DVT prophylaxis (Belch et al. 1981; Cade 1992; Samama et al. 1999 – all cited in Dellinger et al. 2004).
- Stress ulcer prophylaxis (Strothert et al. 1980; Borrero et al. 1985; Bresalier et al. 1987; Cook et al. 1998 – all cited in Dellinger et al. 2004).
- Consideration for limitation of support/treatment escalation (Dellinger et al. 2004).

ACUTE RENAL DYSFUNCTION

Clinical brief

Renal dysfunction is a relatively common and often preventable occurrence in the acutely ill, hospitalised adult. If undetected or untreated this can lead to acute renal failure. Acute renal failure is the final common pathway for a great number of very different diseases and for this reason a comprehensive review of renal failure is not presented here.

Renal dysfunction may present in a number of different ways to the outreach practitioner. Very often this includes a decreased urine output and/or deranged urea and creatinine. This may be an isolated and simple problem such as an obstructed catheter, or it may be a manifestation of a systemic problem such as circulatory shock. In managing this problem it is important to understand why urine output is reduced. The key principles of assessment and timely intervention are of great value in preventing the sequelae of acute renal failure.

Distinguishing the cause of acute renal dysfunction can direct prompt intervention to address the most likely cause or range of contributory factors. This section does not consider specific renal disorders; rather it advocates a broad approach to the patient who is referred to the outreach team with reduced urine output (oliguria). This approach is presented in the algorithm in Figure 4.5 and more expanded considerations for assessment and management are also detailed below.

The key stages outlined in the algorithm are:

* accurately measuring urine output in order to evaluate urine output volumes;
* assessing for and managing simple outflow obstruction (e.g. blocked catheter);
* optimising renal perfusion;
* considering diuretics (after optimising renal perfusion);
* following initial assessment and intervention – formulation of a collaborative management plan including further investigations.

Assessment and investigations – key points

* ABCDE approach including limited but directed history, examination and review of charts.
* Special points in the history:
  * indicators of acute interstitial nephritis (allergic manifestations such as skin rash, non-infectious fever and eosinophilia) in association with drugs implicated in AIN (e.g. penicillin, amoxicillin, cephalosporins, frusemide, thiazides, NSAIDs, allopurinol, captopril (Clive and Cohen 2003));
  * previous/baseline renal function should be given particular attention; previous creatinine and urea may indicate pre-existing renal dysfunction and hence determine whether the presenting dysfunction is acute, chronic or acute on chronic;
  * determine whether there is a likely history of nephrotoxic exposure (e.g. radiocontrast) or ischaemic history (hypotensive episode);
  * other comorbidities and medical history (malignancy. diabetes, cardiac failure, hepatic failure, sepsis, pancreatitis, trauma, burns, volume depletion, recent surgery, crush injuries, myoglobinaemia).
* Physical examination/monitoring:
  * ABCDE approach promptly managing other significant aberrations in vital signs (refer to the sections above for titration of oxygen and fluid challenges);

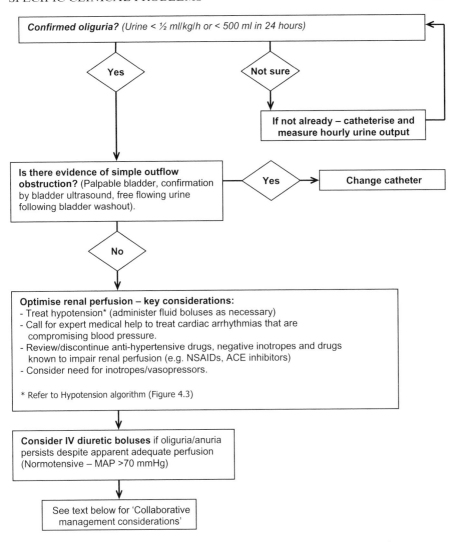

Figure 4.5 The management of oliguria (reduced urine output).

Collaborative management considerations

– Examine the patient fully (A-B-C-D-E and record observations: temperature, pulse, BP, RR, CVP, SpO₂).
– Catheterise if not already catheterised and measure hourly urine volumes.
– Consider the need for urgent expert medical help
– Review recent events and condition changes (from patient, charts and staff); pay particular attention to current/recent drug therapy (or any other administered agent that could cause renal dysfunction).
– Review and request appropriate investigations (FBC, U&E, ABGs, glucose, PO₄, Mg²⁺, Ca²⁺, urine microscopy and culture, blood cultures, CXR, ECG).
– Renal and pelvic ultrasound if there is a risk of ureteric obstruction (e.g. renal calculi surgery).
– Does the patient need renal replacement therapy or expert nephrology review (uraemia, acidosis, hyperkalaemia, fluid overload/pulmonary oedema)?
– Can the patient be managed in their current location (or do they need transfer to critical care or renal unit)?
– Ensure all findings and interventions are documented, that senior medical staff are aware of the patient's condition and that a collaborative plan of care is documented and communicated to the patient, family and multi-disciplinary team.

  ○ determine accurate urine output (by hourly catheter output), past urine trends, vital sign correlations with urine output and accurate fluid volume status.
- Investigations:
  ○ urine tests including bedside specific gravity and 'dipstick' for protein or haem pigments – which may give a rapid indication of pre-renal causes versus intrinsic renal pathology respectively (laboratory: osmolality, electrolytes, creatinine clearance, microscopy and culture, Bence Jones proteins);
  ○ FBC (looking in particular for anaemia (chronic renal dysfunction), leukocytosis (infection/sepsis) and eosinophilia (AIN));
  ○ U&Es – to identify hyperkalaemia which may be the most immediate life-threatening electrolyte imbalance; serial profiles will indicate the rapidity of rise in nitrogenous waste products and the urgency of more advanced intervention such as renal replacement therapy;
  ○ arterial blood gases (to establish pH disturbances and gases exchange alterations);
  ○ LFTs to exclude hepato-renal syndrome (though obvious jaundice would usually be present);
  ○ calcium and phosphate;
  ○ serology (e.g. antinuclear antibodies) if autoimmune has not been ruled out;
  ○ renal ultrasound is a safe and rapid, high-yield procedure in particular for identifying obstructive uropathy (Clive and Cohen 2003).

Management considerations – key points

- Maintain adequate oxygen delivery: oxygen saturation, oxygen carrying capacity – Hb and cardiac output (Sear 2005).
- Supplemental oxygen, or CPAP in the case of significant pulmonary oedema causing hypoxia/dyspnoea.
- Rule out simple catheter obstruction or other causes of obstructive uropathy.
- Correct any pre-renal factors and establish fluid regime that is appropriate to the current volume/hydration status and electrolyte balance and review this regularly (Nowbar and Anderson 2001; Clive and Cohen 2003; Sear 2005).
- Consider diuretics only in the early stages of renal failure and after correction of pre-renal factors and restoration of volume status have proved unsuccessful in improving urine output (Nowbar and Anderson 2001; Sear 2005).
- Review the current drug treatment regime: adjust dose or discontinue as per BNF Appendix 3 and/or seek expert pharmacist advice (in particular

ACE inhibitors and NSAIDs should be avoided) (Clive and Cohen 2003; Sear 2005).

• Ensure that adequate nutrition is provided: refer for expert dietician advice where patients are catabolic or where there are electrolyte derangements (Nowbar and Anderson 2001).
• Management of electrolyte derangement: regulate potassium and phosphate intake and consider pharmacological regimes (calcium resonium or dextrose and insulin for hyperkalaemia; phosphate binders in hyperphosphataemia).
• Refer to critical care consultant or renal dialysis unit and consider the need for renal replacement therapy.

ALTERED LEVEL OF CONSCIOUSNESS

Clinical brief

Consciousness can be defined as a state where one is aware of self and the environment. It is reliant on the interdependent anatomical and physiological components of arousal (wakefulness) and awareness. An altered level of consciousness can result when either or both of these are disturbed through structural lesions or non-structural disorders (Stübgen and Caronna 2001).

Most disorders of consciousness involve impaired arousal and when arousal is affected it is impossible to assess awareness. *Alertness, lethargy, stupor* and *coma* are terms that describe, in the order presented here, the increasing depth of impaired arousal. All acute alterations in consciousness should be regarded as potentially life-threatening emergencies. These present one of the most difficult challenges in clinical management. This is because the number of possible causes is extensive and the time for effective diagnosis and intervention is short (Stübgen and Caronna 2001).

The outreach practitioner may be 'on scene' early in the disease process and may serve as a valuable means of initial assessment, intervention and referral to specialist clinicians. In-hospital transfer for CT scan or to a unit for specialist care and monitoring may also be facilitated by the outreach practitioner. Overall support, education and leadership are a further invaluable contribution that can be made.

This section does not consider specific neurological disorders; rather it advocates a broad approach to the patient who is referred to the outreach team with acutely altered consciousness. This approach is presented in the form of a clinical algorithm (see Figure 4.6) followed by key points on assessment and management. The key stages advocated in the algorithm are as follows.

• Assessing and supporting airway, breathing and circulation.
• Undertaking a rapid neurological assessment.

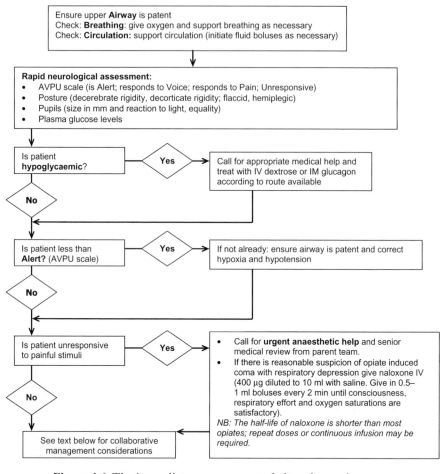

Figure 4.6 The immediate management of altered consciousness.

Collaborative management considerations

– If not already done call for senior medical help.
– Remain with the patient; regularly re-assess ABCDE and intervene as appropriate.
– Establish monitoring (regular GCS, pulse oximetry, temperature and vital signs).
– Review recent events and condition changes (from patient, charts and staff).
– If patient is fitting monitor type and duration of fit activity, protect airway, give oxygen and treat with anticonvulsants, e.g. diazepam 5–10 mg IV or 10 mg PR.
– Is there evidence/history of trauma as a cause of coma (intracranial bleed, contusion)?
– Is there evidence/history of and infective cause for the coma (fever, rash, elevated WBC)?
– Is there evidence/history of metabolic or pharmacological causes of coma (e.g. CNS depressant drugs, hypoglycaemia, electrolyte imbalance, uraemia, hepatic encephalopathy, hypoxia, hypercapnia, profound hypotension)?
– Need for investigations (ABGs, U&Es, glucose, FBC, LFT, Ca^{2+}, Mg^{2+}, blood cultures, ECG, CXR, CT scan).
– Full neurological examination.
– Can the Pt be managed in their current location?
– Is specialist neurology advice needed?
– Ensure all findings and interventions are documented, that senior medical staff are aware of the episode and that a collaborative plan of care is documented and communicated to the patient, family and multi-disciplinary team.
– Review resuscitation status and need to make explicit any limits on treatment escalation.

- Assess for hypoglycaemia, and treat if present.
- If the patient is unresponsive to painful stimuli call for immediate anaesthetic help and senior medical help.
- In patients unresponsive to painful stimuli – if there is a reasonable suspicion of opiate induced coma give naloxone.
- Call for senior medical help and develop a plan for investigation, monitoring and collaborative management.

Assessment and investigations – key points

- Rapid assessment and immediate management should be directed at resuscitation and the limitation of additional brain insult.
- ABCDE approach including limited but directed history, examination and review of charts.
- Rapid neurological assessment including:
  - AVPU scale assessment of responsiveness (**A**lert, responds to **V**oice, responds to **P**ain, **U**nresponsive)
  - pupillary size, symmetry and reaction to light
  - ocular movements
  - motor system assessment (are limb movements appropriate and purposeful or inappropriate and stereotyped, e.g. decerebrate or decorticate rigidity?).
- Ongoing monitoring of GCS, BP, HR, RR, temperature, urine output, SpO_2 at least every 15–30 minutes in the first instance.
- Exclusion and immediate management of metabolic or pharmacological causes of coma:
  - hypoglycaemia – bedside capillary glucose measurement
  - hypothermia – measure core temperature
  - hypoxia – pulse oximetry and arterial blood gases
  - hypotension/hypoperfusion – blood pressure, capillary refill time
  - electrolyte disorders – venous blood for urea and electrolytes
  - opiate overdose, benzodiazepine overdose – prescription chart/drug history.
- Head CT scan to identify any structural lesions causing coma.
- Other blood tests – blood culture, viral titres, liver function tests, coagulation studies, sedative/toxic drug levels, thyroid and adrenal function.
- Urine culture and drugs screen.
- Cerebrospinal fluid microscopy and culture (if infective cause suspected).
- ECG.
- History from family or clinical staff who were witness to the events and circumstances surrounding the change in condition.
- Glasgow coma scale assessment and charting.

- Full neurological examination – however, this should not delay sedation and intubation, resuscitation or transfer for urgent CT scan where these are indicated.

Management considerations – key points

- Rapid management of problems with airway, breathing, oxygenation and circulation (perfusion).
- Rapid seizure control initially with IV benzodiazepines.
- Rapid management/reversal of suspected/identified metabolic or pharmacological causes.
- There should be a low threshold for sedation and intubation in a comatose patient even if respiratory function is initially adequate.
- Ensure measures to reduce rises in intracranial pressure:
  - if intubated – ensure a method of securing the ET tube that allows cephalic venous drainage (tape or tie to allow two fingers of slack);
  - control PaO_2 to >12 kpa (Grant and Andrews 1999);
  - Control $PaCO_2$ to 4.0–4.5 (low normal values) (Grant and Andrews 1999);
  - elevate the head of the bed to at least 15–30° with the head kept in a neutral position (Grant and Andrews 1999);
  - ensure judicious use of IV fluid in those who are not hypovolaemic;
  - avoid hypotonic crystalloid solutions (dextrose and dextrose saline) (Grant and Andrews 1999);
  - aim to keep plasma sodium >140 mmol/l (Grant and Andrews 1999);
  - consider muscle relaxants in the intubated patient where sedation alone is inadequate to control rises in intrathoracic pressure that may cause rises in intracranial pressure (Grant and Andrews 1999).
- Avoid hypoglycaemia and hyperglycaemia (>11 mmol/l) (Grant and Andrews 1999).
- Rapid management of seizure activity.

OTHER COMMON PROBLEMS COMPLICATING CRITICAL ILLNESS

The potential list of conditions that the outreach practitioner may be asked to help assess and manage is vast and dealing with such a list is beyond the scope of this chapter. However, this final section briefly considers three key problems that we have seen which, while they are often not the primary reason for referral to outreach, contribute significantly to the physiological aberration, the severity of the illness or the complexity of assessment and management. For this reason they are included here.

ACUTE PAIN

Despite significant advances in acute pain control over recent years, pain continues to be a confounding factor for many patients including the critically ill (Dolin et al. 2002). Unrelieved pain can result in agitation, inadequate sleep, exhaustion, disorientation and poor compliance with treatment. The associated stress response can involve tachycardia, increased myocardial oxygen demands, hypercoagulability, immunosuppression and catabolism (Lewis et al. 1994; Epstein and Breslow 1999).

Abdominal surgery, pancreatitis and thoracic trauma (with sternal or rib fractures) are examples of cases frequently seen by outreach where good pain control can mean the difference between recovery or deterioration involving pulmonary complications (Desai 1999; Gust et al. 1999). Deterioration often necessitates some form of advanced respiratory therapy including intensive physiotherapy, CPAP and even mechanical ventilation.

The topic of acute pain is vast and is supported by a substantive body of literature. For in-depth consideration of this area the reader is referred to the wider literature. However, the following serve as a few key principles that should underpin outreach practice where pain is a problem.

Pain assessment

• Pain should be systematically and comprehensively assessed. This should include the location, characteristics, aggravating factors, alleviating factors and intensity. Severity should be assessed by the use of a self-report method using one of: visual rating scale, visual analogue scale, numerical rating scale, as appropriate for the individual patient (Jacobi et al. 2002).
• Where patients are unable to communicate regarding their pain, assessment should be informed by subjective and pain-related behaviours (e.g. movement, facial expression, posturing) as well as physiological indicators (e.g. heart rate, blood pressure, respiratory rate) (Jacobi et al. 2002).
• Consistency should be ensured in the method of pain assessment and documentation of severity, to allow evaluation of pain management strategies (Jacobi et al. 2002).

Analgesic strategies

A review of individual analgesics and their individual uses and pharmacology is beyond the cope of this chapter; however, there are some key principles that should underpin analgesic strategies:

• An individual therapeutic plan and goal should be established for patients and communicated to all caregivers to ensure consistency (Jacobi et al. 2002).

- The treatment of choice for severe pain should be opioid analgesics. Where they are indicated morphine, fentanyl and diamorphine are the recommended drugs (Jacobi et al. 2002).
- Fentanyl and diamorphine are preferred for patients with renal insufficiency or haemodynamic instability (Jacobi et al. 2002).
- Non-steroidal anti-inflammatory drugs (NSAIDS) and paracetamol are useful adjuncts to opioid analgesics though close monitoring of renal function and for signs of GI bleeding are recommended (Jacobi et al. 2002).
- The use of regional anaesthetic techniques has many benefits in the management of pain associated with trauma; however, these require specialist knowledge and skills (Elliot 2001).
- Prompt referral should be made to acute pain teams or anaesthetists, according to local service models, when first line measures and analgesics have failed to provide adequate pain control or when it is anticipated that pain control will be complex or difficult due to the nature of injuries, disease processes or comorbidities.

DELIRIUM

Acute 'confusion' in the critically ill is associated with increased morbidity, adverse incidents and even increased mortality (Ely, Guatam, Margolin et al. 2001; Skrobik 2003). This complex clinical problem poses a significant challenge for acute and critical care staff as well as distress to patients and family.

A range of terms have been used to describe the patient with acute psychological disturbance associated with acute/critical illness. However, some consensus is emerging in the literature that the signs and symptoms are consistent with 'delirium' (Truman and Ely 2003).

The essential diagnostic features of delirium are as follows.

- Disturbance of consciousness with reduced ability to focus, sustain or shift attention.
- A change in cognition or development of a perceptual disturbance that is not better accounted for by a pre-existing dementia.
- The disturbance develops over a short period of time and tends to fluctuate.
- There is evidence from history, physical examination or laboratory findings that the disturbance is caused by the physiological consequences of a general medical condition (American Psychiatric Association, DSM-IV 1994).

Within the critical care setting evidence indicates that prevalence may be as high as 80% (Ely, Margolin, Francis et al. 2001). It is thought to be lower in the ward environment but evidence suggests that delirium is unrecognised in

66–84% of patients regardless of their clinical location (Inouye 1994; Rincon et al. 2001; Sanders 2002).

Assessment of the patient with suspected delirium

Identifying the thrashing, agitated paranoid patient with 'hyperactive' delirium is not difficult for clinical staff; however, a further subtype of 'quiet' or 'hypoactive' delirium also occurs. This involves hallucinations and paranoia but not agitation and is associated with a worse prognosis than in non-delirious patients in the ICU (Bergeron et al. 2001). Identifying the hypoactive subtype is more challenging and the use of an assessment tool is advocated.

The Confusion Assessment Method for ICU (CAM-ICU) (Ely, Inouye, Bernard et al. 2001) is a tool that has been developed and validated for use in critical care, including the ventilated ICU patient. According to the CAM-ICU the diagnosis of delirium requires the presence of the following.

1. *Acute onset of mental status changes or a fluctuating course*
   e.g. evidence of an acute change in mental status from the baseline
   - The (abnormal) behaviour fluctuated during the past 24 hours.
   - The sedation scale or coma scale (GCS) fluctuated in the past 24 hours.
2. *Inattention*
   e.g. the patient has difficulty focusing attention
   - There is a reduced ability to maintain and shift attention.
   - The patient cannot successfully complete an attention screening examination (i.e. recall 10 pictures of everyday objects or squeeze hands or nod whenever the letter 'A' is called in a random letter sequence of 10 letters).
   and
3. *Disorganised thinking*
   e.g. if the patient can verbalise, determine whether or not the patient's thinking is disorganised or incoherent, such as rambling or irrelevant conversation, unclear or illogical flow of ideas, or unpredictable switching from subject to subject.

For those unable to verbalise (e.g. tracheostomy), can the patient answer the following four questions correctly?

1. Will a stone float on water?
2. Are there fish in the sea?
3. Does one pound weigh more than two pounds?
4. Can you use a hammer to pound a nail?
   or

4. *Altered level of consciousness*

e.g.

- alert: normal, spontaneously fully aware of environment, interacts appropriately
- vigilant: hyperalert
- lethargic: drowsy but easily aroused, unaware of some elements in the environment, or not spontaneously interacting appropriately with the interviewer; becomes fully aware and appropriately interactive when prodded minimally.

(A kit to implement the CAM-ICU tool in practice, as well as other useful information, is available at: www.icudelirium.org/delirium/index.html.)

Other assessment should involve history, examination and laboratory investigation directed at identifying the underlying aetiology and possible differential diagnosis:

- vital signs (BP, HR, RR, temperature);
- review current drug therapy for possible pharmacological causes (opiates, benzodiazepines);
- evidence of acute withdrawal (from drugs, alcohol);
- evidence of pain;
- focal neurological signs (possibly indicating a structural cause);
- evidence of infection/sepsis as a cause;
- biochemical/endocrine/metabolic causes (haemoglobin, pH, PaO_2, $PaCO_2$, Na, Ca, K, urea, plasma glucose, thiamine, B_{12}, folate, T_4, hepatic failure, porphyria, vascular (hypertensive encephalopathy, systemic lupus erythematosus, vasculitis, polyarteritis nodosa, thromboses) (Ludwig, 1980; Cassem et al. 2001).

Key points on management of delirium

The most important step in delirium treatment is early recognition. Following this, the goals are to improve mental status and minimise risks to the patient (Truman and Ely 2003). To this end the following, while not well supported by research, are suggested.

- Once delirium is detected efforts should be directed towards identifying the underlying aetiology (see above) and addressing any identified causative factors (Truman and Ely 2003).
- Repeated orientation (to place, person and to tubes and lines attached to the patient) and use of a calm voice.
- Cognitive stimulation activities several times per day; this can include cognitive re-assessment such as delirium assessment tools.

- Non-pharmacological sleep protocol, which involves using sedatives/hypnotics only as a last resort; acceptable sleep promoting measures include massages, relaxation tapes, warm drinks, adequate non-sedating analgesia, other usual patient routine/comfort measures.
- Early mobilisation.
- Removing any monitoring, drains or devices that act as physical restraints or cause discomfort.
- Use of devices to facilitate normal sensory functioning (e.g. glasses, hearing aids).
- Reduce dehydration.
- Ensuring adequate analgesia.
- Reducing unnecessary noise and other stimulation.
- Involvement of and reassurance from family.
- Avoidance of benzodiazepines and judicious use of opiates for analgesia (Truman and Ely 2003).
- For the unmanageable patient: use of haloperidol – 2 mg loading dose followed by repeated doses (double the previous dose) every 15–20 minutes while agitation persists. Once the delirium is controlled regular doses (4–6 hourly) should be continued for several days then tapered over several days (Tesar et al. 1985; Tesar and Stern 1988; Jacobi et al. 2002). The interaction with other drugs should be considered and monitoring for side effects, especially those associated with cardiac and sedating effects, should be undertaken.

INADEQUATE NUTRITION

Poor nutrition is common in the UK hospital population (McWhirter and Pennington 1994) leading to increased morbidity and lengths of stay through impaired immunity, tissue healing, muscle strength and psychological drive (Stroud et al. 2003). The detrimental effects of poor nutrition may be of particular significance in the critically ill population due to the severity of their physiological aberration and the risk of negative nitrogen balance through catabolism. The following may serve as useful principles to guide practice.

Nutritional assessment

- A baseline nutritional assessment should be documented for all seriously ill patients (Stroud et al. 2003).
- Commonly available indicators of poor nutrition include (Nompleggi 2003):
  - body mass index <20 (normal range: 20–25 kg/m^2);
  - weight loss >10%; this may be complicated by the presence of oedema – but oedema may in itself be an indicator of significant malnutrition;

o reduced serum proteins (albumin, transferrin, pre-albumin, retinol-binding protein, though hepatic dysfunction and inflammatory processes interfere with normal synthesis);
o reduced serum creatinine and increased creatinine excretion (while measuring urinary excretion of creatinine is advocated in textbooks, this requires accurate 24-hour urine collection; serum creatinine is useful as an indicator of muscle mass; however, renal dysfunction significantly affects creatinine levels and excretion);
o anaemia (low Hb or Hct may accompany chronic poor nutrition, but may be affected by poor iron absorption as well as fluid volume excess or deficit);
o total lymphocyte count (may be decreased in severe debilitating disease but is a relatively late sign of malnutrition).
- In addition to global assessments of nutritional status, measurements of electrolytes (including calcium, magnesium and phosphate) should be undertaken as well as trace elements (e.g. zinc, copper, manganese) (Nompleggi 2003).

Principles related to nutrition

- The provision of adequate nutrition should be a priority in all critically ill patients unless prolongation of life is not in the patient's best interests (Stroud et al. 2003).
- National guidelines recommend that artificial nutrition support is needed when oral intake is absent, or likely to be absent, for a period of >5–7 days (Stroud et al. 2003). Earlier instigation may be needed in malnourished patients and in the critically ill this should commence within the first 24 hours where possible. In all post-surgical patients not tolerating oral intake, enteral tube feeding should be commenced within 1–2 days in the severely malnourished, in 3–5 days in the moderately malnourished, and within seven days in the normally or over-nourished (Stroud et al. 2003).
- The presence of a tracheostomy alone should not prevent oral nutrition unless there is suspicion or evidence of aspiration. If aspiration is suspected, urgent swallowing assessment should be undertaken.
- In the patient who is reluctant to eat, discovering the reasons for this can be very helpful in negotiating a plan of how to improve nutrition.
- Nausea and altered sense of taste are common reasons for loss of appetite. In particular, patients breathing through tracheostomies have reduced taste sensation, at least part of which can be explained by reduced olfactory stimuli.
- Educating the patient about the importance and discipline of eating 'to get well' rather than eating through hunger or pleasure is key.
- Good oral hygiene and analgesia, in the case of painful swallowing or oral lesions, should not be neglected.

- Despite best efforts enteral nutrition may not be possible as the sole, or event supplementary, method of nutrition. Indications for parenteral nutrition include:
  - gut dysfunction (including paralytic ileus and excessive gastric aspirate volumes);
  - where adequate nutrition cannot be achieved safely by the enteral route alone (this may include where there is risk of aspiration or where disease processes result in excessive nutritional demands) (Griffiths 2004).
- Dietetic referral and consultation should be initiated early in order to establish appropriate nutritional goals and strategies.

Disclaimer

This chapter is intended as a guide and the reader is encouraged to act at all times in accordance with local protocols and clinical judgement. The authors take no responsibility for any actions that practitioners take as a result of reading this chapter.

REFERENCES

American College of Chest Physicians/Society of Critical Care Medicine Consensus Conference Committee (1992) American College of Chest Physicians/Society of Critical Care Medicine Consensus Conference: Definitions for sepsis and organ failure and guidelines for the use of innovative therapies in sepsis. *Critical Care Medicine* 20: 864–74.

American College of Surgeons Committee on Trauma (1997) *American Trauma Life Support for Doctors.* Chicago: American College of Surgeons.

American Psychiatric Association (1994) *Diagnostic and Statistical Manual of Mental Disorders* 4th edn (DSM-IV). Washington: American Psychiatric Association.

American Society of Anaesthesiologists (1996) Practice Guidelines for Blood Component Therapy. A report by the American Society of Anaesthesiologists Taskforce on Blood Component Therapy. *Anaesthesiology* 84: 732–47.

Annane D, Sebille V, Charpentier C et al. (2002) Effect of treatment with low doses of hydrocortisone and fludrocortisone on mortality of patients with septic shock. *Journal of the American Medical Association* 288: 862–71.

Bergeron N, Dubois MJ, Dumont M et al. (2001) Intensive care delirium screening checklist: Evaluation of a new screening tool. *Intensive Care Medicine* 27: 859–64.

Bernard GR, Artigas A, Brigham KL et al. (1994) Report of the American-European Consensus Conference on ARDS: Definitions, mechanisms, relevant outcomes and clinical trial co-ordination. *Intensive Care Medicine* 20(3): 225–32.

Bernard GR, Vincent JL, Laterre PF et al. (2001) Efficacy and safety of recombinant human activated protein C for severe sepsis. *New England Journal of Medicine* 344: 699–709.

British Thoracic Society (2001) Guidelines for the management of community acquired pneumonia. *Thorax* 56 Suppl. IV.

British Thoracic Society (2002) (British Thoracic Society Standards of Care Committee) Non-invasive ventilation in acute respiratory failure. *Thorax* 57: 192–211.

British Thoracic Society & Scottish Intercollegiate Guideline Network (2004) *British Guideline on the Management of Asthma.* London: British Thoracic Society & Scottish Intercollegiate Guidelines Network.

Cassem NH, Lopez GA, Bleck TP (2001) Acute and subacute psychiatric disorders. In JE Parrillo and RP Dellinger (eds) *Critical Care Medicine: Principles of Diagnosis and Management in the Adult* 2nd edn. pp. 1586–96. St Louis: Mosby.

Celli BR, Snider GL, Heffner J et al. (1995) Standards for the diagnosis and care of patients with chronic obstructive pulmonary disease (Official statement of the American Thoracic Society, medical section of the American Lung Association). *American Review of Respiratory Disease* 152 (Suppl). S72–120.

Clive DM, Cohen AJ (2003) Acute renal failure in the intensive care unit. In RS Irwin and JM Rippe (eds) *Irwin and Rippe's Intensive Care Medicine* 5th edn. pp. 889–911. Philadelphia: Lippincott, Williams & Wilkins.

Connaughton M (2001) *Evidence-Based Manual of Coronary Care Management.* London: Churchill Livingstone.

Dellinger RP, Carlet JM, Masur H et al. (2004) Surviving sepsis campaign guidelines for management of severe sepsis and septic shock. *Critical Care Medicine* 32(3): 858–73.

Desai PM (1999) Pain management and pulmonary dysfunction. *Critical Care Clinics* 15: 151–66.

Dolin S et al. (2002) Effectiveness of acute postoperative pain management: I. Evidence from published data. *British Journal of Anaesthesia* 89: 409–23

Elliot J M (2001) Regional anaesthesia in trauma. *Trauma* 3: 161–74.

Ely EW, Gautam S, Margolin R et al. (2001) The impact of delirium in the intensive care unit on hospital length of stay. *Intensive Care Medicine* 27: 1892–1900.

Ely EW, Inouye SK, Bernard GR et al. (2001) Delirium in mechanically ventilated patients. Validity and reliability of the confusion assessment method for the intensive care unit (CAM-ICU). *Journal of the American Medical Association* 286: 2703–10.

Ely EW, Margolin R, Francis J et al. (2001) Evaluation of delirium in critically ill patients: validation of the confusion assessment method for the intensive care unit (CAM-ICU). *Critical Care Medicine* 29: 1370–9.

Epstein J, Breslow MJ (1999) The stress response of critical illness. *Critical Care Clinics* 15:17–33.

Forrester J, Diamond G, Swan H (1977) Correlative classification of clinical and haemodynamic function after acute myocardial infarction. *American Journal of Cardiology* 39: 137–54.

Grant IS, Andrews JD (1999) ABC of intensive care neurological support. *British Medical Journal* 319: 110–13.

Green C, Dinnes J, Takeda A, Shepherd J, Hartwell D, Cave C et al. (2005) Clinical effectiveness and cost effectiveness of drotrecogin alpha (activated) (Xigris®) for the treatment of severe sepsis in adults: a systematic review and economic evaluation. *Health Technology Assessment* 9(11).

Griffiths RD (2004) *Which Critically Ill Patients should receive TPN?* Intensive Care Society.

Gust R, Pecher S, Gust A et al. (1999) Effect of patient-controlled analgesia on pulmonary complications after coronary artery-bypass grafting. *Critical Care Medicine* 27: 2218–23.

Hollenburg SM, Kavinsky CJ, Parillo JE (1999) Cardiogenic shock. *Annals of Internal Medicine* 131(47).

Hollenburg SM, Parillo JE (2001) Cardiogenic shock. In JE Parrillo and RP Dellinger (eds) *Critical Care Medicine: Principles of Diagnosis and Management in the Adult* 2nd edn. pp. 421–36. St Louis: Mosby.

Inouye SK (1994) The dilemma of delirium: clinical and research controversies regarding diagnosis and evaluation of delirium in hospitalized elderly medical patients. *American Journal of Medicine* 97: 278–88.

Jacobi J et al. (2002) Clinical practice guidelines for the sustained use of sedatives and analgesics in the critically ill adult. *Critical Care Medicine* 30(1): 119–41.

Jimenez MF, Marshall JC (2001) Source control in the management of sepsis. *Intensive Care Medicine* 27: S49–62.

Killip T, Kimball JT (1967) Treatment of myocardial infarction in a coronary care unit: a two year experience with 250 patients. *American Journal of Cardiology* 20: 457.

Kumar A, Parrillo JE (2001) Shock: Classification, pathophysiology and approach to management. In JE Parrillo and RP Dellinger (eds) *Critical Care Medicine: Principles of Diagnosis and Management in the Adult* 2nd edn. pp. 371–420. St Louis: Mosby.

Levy MM. Fink MP, Marshall JC, Abraham E, Angus D, Cook D et al. (2003) SCCM/ESICM/ACCP/ATS/SIS International Sepsis Definitions Conference. *Critical Care Medicine* 31(4): 1250–6.

Lewis KS, Whipple JK, Michael KA et al. (1994) Effect of analgesic treatment on the physiological consequences of acute pain. *American Journal of Hospital Pharmacy* 51:1539–54.

Ludwig AM (1980) *Principles of Clinical Psychiatry.* New York: The Free Press.

McWhirter JP, Pennington CR (1994) Incidence and recognition of malnutrition in hospital. *British Medical Journal* 308(6934): 945–8.

Madais JE (2000) Killip and Forrester Classifications – should they be abandoned, kept, re-evaluated, or modified? *Chest* 117: 1223–6.

National Institute for Clinical Excellence (2004) *Chronic Obstructive Pulmonary Disease: Management of Chronic Obstructive Pulmonary Disease in Adults in Primary and Secondary Care.* Clinical Guideline 12. National Institute for Clinical Excellence.

Niederman MS (2001) Pneumonia: considerations in the critically ill patient. In JE Parrillo and RP Dellinger (eds) *Critical Care Medicine: Principles of Diagnosis and Management in the Adult* 2nd edn. pp. 780–807. St Louis: Mosby.

Nompleggi DJ (2003) Basic principles of nutrition support in the intensive care unit. In RS Irwin and JM Rippe (eds) *Irwin and Rippe's Intensive Care Medicine* 5th edn. pp. 2053–7. Philadelphia: Lippincott, Williams & Wilkins.

Nowbar S, Anderson RJ (2001) Acute renal failure. In JE Parrillo, RP Dellinger (eds) *Critical Care Medicine: Principles of Diagnosis and Management in the Adult* 2nd edn, pp. 1133–56. St Louis: Mosby.

Rincon HG, Granados M, Unutzer J et al. (2001) Prevalence, detection, and treatment of anxiety, depression and delirium in the adult critical care unit. *Psychosomatics* 42: 391–6.

Rivers E, Nguyen B, Havstad S et al. (2001) Early goal-directed therapy in the management of severe sepsis and septic shock. *New England Journal of Medicine* 345: 1368–77.

Ruch V (1999) Pulmonary disorders. In A Gawlinski and D Hamwi (eds) *Acute Care Nurse Practitioner: Clinical Curriculum and Certification Review.* pp. 16–135. Philadelphia: WB Saunders Co.

Sanders AB (2002) Missed delirium in older emergency department patients: a quality-of-care problem. *Annals of Emergency Medicine* 39: 338–41.

Sear JW (2005) Kidney dysfunction in the postoperative period. *British Journal of Anaesthesia* 95(1): 20–32.

Skrobik Y (2003) An overview of delirium in the critical care setting. *Geriatrics & Aging* 6(10): 30–5.

Stroud M, Duncan H, Nightingale J (2003) Guidelines for enteral feeding in the adult hospital patient. *Gut* 52 (Suppl VII): 1–12.

Stübgen JP, Caronna JJ (2001) Coma. In JE Parrillo and RP Dellinger (eds) *Critical Care Medicine: Principles of Diagnosis and Management in the Adult* 2nd edn. pp. 1259–77. St Louis: Mosby.

Tesar GE, Murray GB, Cassem NH (1985) Use of haloperidol for acute delirium in intensive care setting. *Journal of Clinical Psychopharmacology* 5: 344–7.

Tesar GE, Stern TA (1988) Rapid tranquilization of the agitated intensive care unit patient. *Journal of Intensive Care Medicine* 3:195–201.

Truman B, Ely EW (2003) Monitoring delirium in critically ill patients: using the confusion assessment method for the intensive care unit. *Critical Care Nurse* 23(2): 25–35.

Weinstein MP, Reller LP, Murphy JR et al. (1983) The clinical significance of positive blood cultures: A comprehensive analysis of 500 episodes of bacteremia and fungemia in adults. I Laboratory and epidemiological observations. *Review of Infectious Diseases* 5: 35–53.

5 Sharing critical care skills

LEE CUTLER, KATHRYN WARREN AND RINKY INGLIS

INTRODUCTION

It has been assumed that failures in recognition and care of the critically ill patient in acute ward areas, what has been described as 'sub-optimal care' (McQuillan et al. 1998; McGloin et al. 1999), are at least in part related to failures in education and training for healthcare professionals. The chapter will explore the challenges these failures pose for outreach practitioners as well as approaches aimed at addressing these issues. While the chapter discusses policy as well as theoretical and empirical literature, it is informed mainly by real-life experience gained in the process of striving to improve the care of the critically ill in the acute hospital setting through the facilitation of learning. A broad approach to sharing critical care skills within the acute hospital is discussed and examples from the authors' practice are used throughout.

The chapter is followed by a case study which demonstrates how the *'RAMSI Course'* (Recognition and Management of the Seriously Ill) used state-of-the-art technology in clinical education for multi-disciplinary critical care staff.

BACKGROUND

There is substantial literature, including research, policy and commentary, regarding the background of critical care outreach and its role in sharing critical care skills, including education of multi-disciplinary practitioners. It is beyond the scope of this chapter to give a representative overview of this literature here; however, several salient points are evident.

First, in the late 1990s various studies provided evidence that there were failures in the care of acutely ill adults on general wards. These included failure to make and record basic clinical observations, to recognise when these were abnormal and to treat promptly and/or call for more expert help in managing these patients.

Critical Care Outreach. Edited by Lee Cutler and Wayne Robson.
Copyright 2006 by John Wiley & Sons Ltd.

Some indicative literature includes a study by McGloin et al. (1997) who found that 65% of cardiac arrests were preventable, whereas only one-third of cardiac arrests were unavoidable. McQuillan et al. (1998), in exploring this further, identified that this 'sub-optimal care' was related to oversights in airway, breathing and circulation problems, including failures to recognise, coordinate and prioritise the delivery of potentially stabilising care. While McQuillan et al.'s study was criticised by some (Gorard 1999) for its failure to define 'sub-optimal care' adequately, the volume and credibility of other supporting literature gave rise to the realisation among those outside the fields of acute and critical care that patients were not receiving the care that they needed. Within critical care this had been realised some time ago by many. Numerous studies predating McQuillan et al. (1998) had shown a failure to refer or admit critically ill ward patients to high dependency units (HDU) or intensive care units (ICU) where they could receive 'critical care' (Metcalf and MacPherson 1995; Crighton and Winter 1997; Wallis et al. 1997).

All this came at a time when national critical care capacity problems were making headlines in the media. In 1999 the Audit Commission published their report, *Critical to Success* (Audit Commission 1999) which concluded:

> critical care is of life-saving importance (but) services are fragmented, expensive and under pressure. And while there is a strong database about the illnesses of patients, there has been a dearth of useful management information about critical care resources, the treatments given and their effectiveness. (Audit Commission 1999, p. 3)

In 2000 a national strategy aimed at addressing the problems identified in critical care was published in the form of *Comprehensive Critical Care* (Department of Health 2000). Three remedial themes were evident within this, as well as other documents (McQuillan et al. 1998; Audit Commission 1999; NCEPOD 1999). These were:

- professional education and development for healthcare staff;
- management of services and resources within trusts and between trusts;
- policies and an evidence base for practice through audit and information gathering.

More recent publications continue to emphasise these themes (DoH 2005; NCEPOD 2005).

The focus of this chapter is the first of these. Critical care outreach is seen as a key player in sharing the expertise and skills that could help to improve the care of those who become critically ill outside the walls of critical care units (DoH 2000, 2005). Specifically, outreach teams should

> share critical care skills in wards and the community ensuring enhancement of training opportunities and skills practice and to use information gathered from the ward and community to improve critical care services for patients and relatives. (DoH 2000, p. 15)

AN APPROACH TO SHARING CRITICAL CARE SKILLS

The difficulties associated with facilitating learning on a hospital-wide scale are significant. This is one of the major challenges facing critical care outreach today. Time and effort need to be focused on areas of priority while at the same time initiating long-term change on a wide scale. Education both complements and is supported by experienced critical care practitioners' role modelling and guidance in practice.

The following sections discuss some of the important goals and areas of work around the sharing of critical care skills. We have shared our approach, which may offer a useful perspective for readers who are asking themselves, 'How do other outreach practitioners go about this work?' Some of the points made may seem obvious but one of the principles of this book and of our chapter is to share our experiences, our thoughts and our successes in order that the importance of the seemingly everyday elements of our role are validated in the text. Examples are given in an attempt to clarify the practical application of the approach and give meaning to the discussion.

IDENTIFYING 'TARGET' AREAS

The first task for critical care staff in sharing their expertise is to identify and describe unacceptable areas or themes within clinical care that can significantly affect the processes and outcomes of caring for the critically ill. It is important to state, in understandable terms, the importance of the area of practice and how this may affect care and outcomes.

It is useful to begin by describing the problem as it is perceived. This often involves anecdotes and experiences from our daily practice. Such anecdotes can often be very powerful (Intensive Care Society 2002). It could simply be that one of us is having a 'bad day' or, for example, it is part of coming to terms with the stark difference between ICU and the ward. However, when similar stories are shared by different team members, and when clinical incident reports or feedback from other practitioners point to failures in care, this highlights areas or themes in care that need to be targeted with intervention, This may often include education even if other measures are also needed.

A principle we believe is important to employ is that one should 'seek first to understand, then to be understood' (Covey 1989). This may mean that further audit or investigation is undertaken, but the important point here is to understand the situation and the 'problem' fully before deciding on, and attempting to argue the case for, a solution. One such solution may focus on or utilise an element of education. However, in our experience, knowledge or skill deficit alone is rarely the problem and education alone is rarely the solution.

It has been advocated that 'individual organisations should undertake education and training needs analyses to identify particular areas of risk' (Modernisation Agency 2003, p. 13). Our initial work in practice involved undertaking a range of activities to enhance our understanding of the problems we perceived. Local audit (Heap et al. 1999) gave a broad overview at the expense of in-depth understanding. This included staff surveys and scoping work to identify critical care skills deficit.

In our hospital-wide survey of nurses, across clinical grades, 79% identified recognition of critical illness as a priority area for improvement of their skills. This relates to the question most commonly asked by ward staff, 'What am I looking for?' (Daffurn et al. 1994; Cioffi 2000): 89% of nurses thought that an early warning system was essential in helping with the recognition of critical illness by themselves as well as by medical staff; 95% of the nurses requested clinical support, specifically with tracheostomies. Other interventions and equipment were also seen as key areas where skill enhancement was needed. Our survey findings were echoed in the literature of the time (Haines and Coad 2001) and provided evidence that led to the successful establishment of a critical care outreach team (Murch and Warren 2001). Coad and Haines (1999) reported on the critical care learning needs of acute ward nurses. The source of the data informing their report was an audit of previous advice given to ward staff as well as discussions with senior nurse managers and ward managers. Reported areas identified for support included:

- haemodynamic assessment
- inotropes/drug therapy
- medical equipment
- central venous pressure (CVP) lines
- fluid and electrolyte imbalance and therapy
- management of tracheostomies
- high flow oxygen therapy
- continuous positive airway pressure (CPAP)
- arterial blood gases.

A further problem area perceived by the ward nurses in our audit was communication between nursing and medical staff. One nurse wrote: 'make them come to the wards and act'. Discussion with nurses from diverse clinical areas and specialties as well as evidence from literature show that this issue has a long international history (Stein 1967; Benner et al. 1996). It has also been argued that effective communication between nurses and doctors is part of expert practice (Benner 1984) and in particular the elements of 'getting appropriate and timely responses from physicians' and 'presenting a case'. Clearly the term 'sharing skills' does not accurately represent the teaching–learning processes that are required for the development of expertise in this domain of professional practice. However, there are some general principles and good habits that can be adopted which can significantly improve communication and teamwork.

Process mapping also worked well in giving us a greater understanding of the detail. One example was about what happens when abnormal observations are recorded. Another useful piece of information came from closely watching the daily routine on acute wards, including exactly how long it takes to record a set of observations and how long the additional task of adding up the scores for a track and trigger tool would take. This gives meaning to the statement made above about understanding things in detail before presenting a case for a solution. Knowing that the additional task takes *fifteen seconds* is a powerful piece of information when it comes to arguing your case.

Research undertaken (Cutler 2002) facilitated a deeper understanding of the cultural context in which critical care skills would be learned and practised and the dilemmas for the nurses. While the understanding arrived at through qualitative studies may not translate directly into 'Do X instead of Y and the result will be . . .', it does allow what have been called 'fuzzy generalisations' (Bassey 1999) to be made. These inform us of the human side of complex, clinical situations as well as building a bridge between critical care and the wards through understanding the culture 'out there'.

In some cases there is evidence from a range of sources that an issue is affecting care across healthcare institutions. One such example is making and recording clinical observations, as well as appropriate responses to abnormal observations. This is a particularly salient example since it appears to be a national problem (McQuillan et al. 1998; McGloin et al. 1999; NCEPOD 1999; Neale et al. 2001). It is a problem that has been much more difficult to address than one might imagine. This is evidenced by the fact that, despite wide acknowledgement of the value of observations and significant activity over a period of several years, it is still a weak link in the chain of identification and care of the critically ill (NCEPOD 2005). The official national outreach perspective is that:

> Diligent, skilled monitoring of patients physiological vital signs, with timely and appropriate response to abnormalities, are fundamental to the pre-emptive care of patients with established or potential critical illness. (Modernisation Agency 2003, p. 15)

By the mid to late 1990s a culture had developed within which observations seemed to have reduced status within the daily work of acute ward nurses. They had been delegated to healthcare support workers, and some may argue that the problem was compounded by the move into an era of what might be called 'hands-free' observations. The result of this has been to mechanise the process. Counting respirations, along with the pulse, somehow was no longer included as routine because pulse rates were automatically displayed with the BP and oxygen saturations.

Like many our initial audit, in the early days of outreach, found that observations were incomplete, inaccurate and in some cases abnormality was completely ignored. There was often a failure to respond to abnormal observations with intelligent nursing or medical care. This was not acceptable and things had to change on a wide scale since observations are the first line of objective surveillance for deterioration in patients' condition.

Unlike clinical observations, in some instances the areas of concern identified may be of a more local nature. We have seen particular issues on particular wards and have heard of other similarly local examples in our conversations with outreach colleagues across the country. On occasions these local issues arise because a particular ward deals with specific clinical problems, monitoring or intervention too infrequently to maintain their skills. On other occasions a large influx of new nurses on a ward dilutes the skill mix and the team requires support until they have gained experience and local knowledge and skills. On other occasions the cause of problems is indiscernible and despite our best efforts we never really get to the root of the problem but employ an educational approach in the interim and things improve. Perhaps this is partly through learning and partly through the 'Hawthorne effect' (Roethlisberger and Dickinson 1939) as outreach takes an interest and highlights inadequacies in care.

EDUCATIONAL IMPLICATIONS

The next part of the approach we advocate is to consider the educational implications of the 'problem'. The greater the understanding of the problem the better the ability of the educator to draw conclusions and plan an appropriate educational strategy. A thorough understanding of the 'problem' should stimulate critical reflection on the overall desired outcomes of addressing the problem, and whether these can be achieved through education alone or in combination with other strategies. In many cases clearly what is required is behaviour change. But achieving this in many instances will take more than increasing understanding, reasoning skills or practical skills. Human beings are complex creatures, who are habitual and who do not always act rationally. As healthcare professionals working in the modern NHS their actions are affected by complex organisations and inherent cultures. The reality is that just because someone 'knows that . . .' it does not mean that this knowledge will be a dominant factor affecting how they behave in a given situation. Understanding people and how change can effectively be managed within and between groups is often what is needed. Acknowledging this at an early stage allows effective planning to bring about the desired behaviour change from many angles. Furthermore it acknowledges the limitations of education and will not leave the teachers feeling that they have done a bad job if people do not behave differently following education.

Being able to describe learning outcomes or competencies is very useful. A recent review of critical care services advised that 'Education and Training are fundamental to support the workforce and should be . . . matched to competencies' (DoH 2005, p. 17). Competencies can focus and guide efforts to facilitate learning. They may also need revision and compromise when the practicalities of achieving the level of learning are critically considered. But they serve as a useful starting point allowing activity to be goal directed and for audit and evaluation to be undertaken against standards. While many in the outreach and critical care community have developed local competency frameworks leading to a rich diversity in practice, national competencies linked to existing frameworks will also be implemented in future (DoH 2005).

The most challenging part of the approach advocated here for some, especially those who are not qualified or very experienced teachers, is to consider what form of educational activity or approach will best achieve the learning outcomes or competencies in the group of individuals concerned. Clearly practical skills do not lend themselves to mainly theoretically based classroom sessions, and complex concepts in physiology, disease and therapy require some 'chalk and talk' even if heavily supplemented by practical examples, case studies and scenarios to work through.

There is no one best way of facilitating learning, and in reality different people learn best using different approaches which suit their learning style. The wisdom of Carl Rogers always comes to mind when this point is discussed in our teams:

> Teaching, in my estimation, is a vastly overrated function . . . I see the facilitation of learning as the aim of education. (Rogers 1969)

Rogers's theory was that education should be learner-centred. However, it is probably the case that Rogers greatly underestimated his ability as a teacher. It is not our intent to discourage teaching in the traditional sense, rather to encourage a range of activities that stimulate, challenge, motivate. Most importantly they should involve the learner as an active participant in their learning rather than encouraging passive reception (Brookfield 1986; Sotto 1994). The reality is that education within hospitals takes place in the context of limited time and resources and has to get a message across to the many by the few. For this reason teachers should have a whole range of approaches that can be widely used and allow diversity in learning. Examples we have used in practice include:

- the seminar/lecture where information is presented and discussed;
- the discussion of cases/experiences within a group where learning comes from real-life experiences and observations to give the theory meaning;
- directed learning packages focused on theoretical principles;
- guided learning/worksheets that require clinical, patient-centred activity;
- skill stations/workshops where practical skills can be demonstrated, practised and supervised;
- software and computer-based interactive learning packages that give the learner flexibility and options in their learning including self-tests;
- simulation and role play in which learners put into practice what they are able to do in a safe, non-threatening and supportive atmosphere;
- quizzes, crosswords – portable self-tests and memory joggers;
- suggested reading – this guides the learner towards material that is appropriate to the learning task at hand.

Probably the most useful thing the educator can do is to become confident enough to select an approach or approaches according to the needs of the learners and the topic or skill to be learned. This means not having a favourite way of teaching or particular habits, but rather being adaptable and learner centred. Confidence comes with experience, but experience does not mean repetition of the same thing in the same way with the same types of learners. It means varying your activity, your methods and your audience. This may sound simple but it is often espoused and not practised.

BARRIERS TO LEARNING

Another consideration in achieving the educational goals is the barriers that stand in the way. Often these are to do with organisational constraints such as limited time to attend teaching sessions. Time constraints related to competing demands of the role also affect our ability as educators to plan, coordinate, facilitate and evaluate educational sessions or programmes. While time to attend may not be seen as a barrier to learning in the broader educational literature, the reality is that for healthcare professionals in the NHS this is increasingly a barrier.

Pragmatic solutions to these issues need to be found. A good way to start is to make a list of all the regular teaching programmes that are already ongoing within the hospital or trust. This gives the opportunity to save time and effort by taking advantage of the fact that someone else (usually administrative staff) undertakes tasks associated with organising the sessions. These tasks include booking a venue, organising a list of those who can attend, evaluating the session, as well as ensuring that there will be enough attending to make it worth while delivering the session. This will save you valuable time and ensure that you meet all new recruits to the hospital and get across your key messages. Because attendance at many of these sessions is mandatory, lack of time to attend is not such an issue.

Examples of maximising this kind of opportunity for teaching include:

- building critical care outreach key training into mandatory update days/ sessions;
- securing a slot on induction programmes for junior medical staff;
- securing a slot on induction days for newly appointed/newly registered nurses;
- securing a slot on other rolling programmes that exist within the hospital or individual wards or directorates, such as directorate audit meetings for raising awareness of issues.

Cultural aspects also serve to complicate the changes we wish to achieve through teaching. These aspects include beliefs and values within teams and professional groups. At the risk of making broad generalisations, examples we have seen are that surgical nurses have generally been more concerned with accurate fluid balance than have medical nurses, while medical nurses may pay more attention to respiratory rate than surgical nurses. Influencing culture is difficult especially in the short term, but education is one way of bringing about cultural change in the long term. However, this requires pressure and/or support from other angles as well. A key point is that the cultural context in which learners are to apply their new knowledge is an important determinant of the success they will achieve in application (Cutler 2002). One implication of this is that education away from the bedside needs to be reinforced by support, encouragement and role modelling back at the bedside. One of the greatest strengths of outreach is that it allows expert critical care professionals to demonstrate best practice. No amount of 'telling' has the power of observing an expert at work.

A final point is about the individual's perception of their learning needs. While the organisational and cultural factors have been briefly considered above we have said nothing of the individual. The individual factors that can affect learning include lack of support and recognition as well as lack of awareness and understanding of future expectations and resistance to change (Gibson 1998). However, in addition we have repeatedly seen one in particular that is worthy of at least brief consideration here. In our experience, in addition to organisational and cultural factors, the learner needs to appreciate their need to learn. This raises the issue of what Benner et al. (1996, p. 194) call 'secondary ignorance'; that is 'They do not know what they do not know, and they may not see a situation or know when action is needed.' This is perhaps evident, one could argue, from some of the rather general topics that are indicated by those who responded to our survey of nurses as well as in published literature (Coad and Haines 1999). Such a phenomenon essentially means that asking ward nurses what they need to know about critical care may not yield specific, valid or reliable results. Also offering to teach about a given topic may receive the response from some that they 'do not need to know about that' or 'already know'. It is not to say that individuals cannot make valid judgements about their learning needs, but we have found that presenting audit findings or case studies from practice gives an opportunity to challenge what individuals think they know and challenge their opinions of what is relevant and what is not. After all, one could argue that the purpose of education is to challenge – how we respond to the challenge is the great unknown and unpredictable element of adult learning.

EVALUATION

This is multi-faceted and can involve many approaches. Evaluation is about the achievement of the learner and the success of the teacher. We are usually concerned with three questions:

1. Has the learning experience been positive for the learner?
2. Have the learning outcomes been achieved?
3. Has the learning been applied in practice?

Answers to the first question are usually gleaned from feedback during the educational activity and from anonymous written student evaluations. Education is not simply about keeping the learners happy but it is widely acknowledged that individuals learn most when the experience is positive for them.

Much has been written about the attributes of teachers that help individuals to learn. These include: being clear and enthusiastic, being excellent communicators, a willingness to use a variety of approaches, concern for the learner, striving to share knowledge and being knowledgeable on the subject. The only attribute actually found to inhibit learning is being critical of the learner (Rogers 1969; Brookfield 1986; Sotto 1994).

Answering the latter two questions is the 'Holy Grail' in education, more so for the final question. The literature reveals that very few studies have demonstrated a link between post-registration education and clinical outcomes (Jordan 2000). Only 118 out of 2000 papers on professional education for healthcare professionals assessed patient outcomes (Grant and Stanton 1998). In Oxman's (1994) systematic review of 102 trials of interventions designed to improve the performance of healthcare professionals, only 12 studies evaluated the impact of educational initiatives on professional performance; Oxman concluded that their effect was modest.

Despite this there are some fundamental characteristics of programmes of learning that have been found to correlate with successful education for practice. These should be central to the way evaluation is undertaken, as well as how teaching/learning activities are developed. These characteristics were first described by Rogers and Shoemaker (1971) in relation to the adoption of innovations in practice. Francke et al. (1995) later generalised these concepts to education and empirical study supports their value in this area (Heick 1981; Cervero 1985; Ferrell 1988; Sheperd 1995; Jordan and Hughes 1998; Jordan 1999).

The characteristics:

- *Compatibility* – is the degree to which the programme content is compatible with the needs of the practitioner and the organisation.
- *Relative advantage* – is the degree to which the learned material is perceived as better than that which it supersedes.
- *Practical applicability* – is the extent to which learned material can be applied, trialled and experimented with in the real life of practice.

Ensuring that evaluation is structured around these characteristics makes sense in theoretical and practical terms. Evaluation may ask students for verbal or written feedback about how they rate the learning in ways which relate to 'compatibility' and 'relative advantage'. Evaluation of learning may also involve formal or informal testing, such as how well learners cope with tasks, questions or scenarios following education.

Perhaps the best indicator of 'practical applicability' is how practice changes. One example of an educational outcome that is increasingly seen in practice is the 'ABCDE' approach to conducting the primary survey of a patient. An objective indicator that this has been applied in practice is medical case notes where, in our experience, this approach structures the text of doctors' record-keeping with increasing frequency.

SUSTAINABILITY AND LONG-TERM CHANGE

While one could argue that education is by its very nature proactive and focused on the future, what has been discussed so far might be considered a rather reactive approach. Ways of identifying and addressing existing problems have in general been the focus so far. However, it is important to acknowledge that if long-term change is to be achieved and if the problems seen in critical care are to be prevented in future then long-term, sustainable, change needs to take place on a national scale. We need to ensure that the healthcare professionals of tomorrow enter practice with better critical care skills than current staff gained from their undergraduate and pre-registration training.

Support for long-term change needs to come through a variety of activities, many of which have been highlighted in a range of strategic documents regarding critical care services. These are briefly discussed here.

Long-term change requires support from professional bodies in the standards they set as well as through academic programmes that prepare individuals for practice prior to professional registration. It has been recommended that pre-registration programmes support students in developing the competencies required for the assessment of acutely ill patients – which involves a mix of theoretical taught content as well as appropriate clinical experience and support through placements and clinical mentorship (DoH 2001). Outreach nurses should strive to ensure that their views shape future curricula in nursing with regard to critical care skills.

For medical staff it is equally important that their training in critical care skills begins at a very early stage. National professional organisations, Royal Colleges and professional regulatory bodies have a role in indicating minimum standards of patient care and clinical competence (Modernisation Agency 2003). Frameworks have been suggested, and are being implemented, which introduce basic assessment of the seriously ill and resuscitation skills in early years of undergraduate medical training. This is then reinforced and expanded throughout undergraduate year. As doctors then graduate and progress through foundation years into specialist career training more advanced courses such as ALERT and ALS (Advanced Life Support) are built in.

A theme running through this training is the timely identification and management of the seriously ill patient. Even the curriculum of the Advanced Life Support course, traditionally a course aimed at resuscitating those already in arrest, now has a major focus on preventing cardiac arrest. Such changes will reinforce and be reinforced by concepts and skills that healthcare professionals will be encouraged to learn throughout their professional education.

These changes in training and preparation for professional practice, as well as evaluation of outcomes from these, need to be guided by explicit key competencies for critical care. However, it is important that competencies are seen as explicit descriptions of areas of role and professional practice rather than accurately representing professional practice which is more complex, holistic and integrated than can be represented in competencies (Cutler 2000).

The 'Skills for Health' initiative leading on from the invaluable work of Kim Manley will result in a range of competencies for all members of the team who care for critically ill patients (DoH 2005). The development and dissemination of these and the establishment of appropriate models of work-based education and training, especially across the nursing workforce, are seen as a key target in ensuring the long-term change required (DoH 2001). Outreach practitioners are in a key position to inform these competencies and how they are interpreted and implemented, as well as how support for the associated learning is provided. A vital part of this is ensuring that all nurses working in critical care, wards and departments have access to competency-based education and training to ensure fitness for purpose (DoH 2001).

These are not simply matters for individual trusts or hospitals, they often require that a strategic review of funding for, access to and provision of education and training is undertaken. Recommendations for such reviews to take place have been made (DoH 2001). The role of outreach in this regard is again to ensure that their view and information they may have about levels of critical care skill and training in acute ward areas inform debates around these issues at trust level. This can then inform the picture that strategic health authorities have of local education needs.

The responsibilities for achieving long-term sustainable change are spread across clinical, educational and strategic spheres. However, the achievement of these requires that decisions are informed by what is happening at grass roots. Critical care outreach staff are well placed to inform these processes and impress upon those working at more strategic levels the implications for the future. This in essence comes down to the sustainability of critical care services and proactive and preventive strategies rather than 'fire fighting'.

The essence of sustainability also lies in the balance between empowerment of ward staff and ownership by critical care, and in investment in the future as well as an ability to identify and deal promptly with problems in care.

CONCLUSION

Sharing critical care skills with multi-disciplinary staff throughout acute care areas is a key role for outreach practitioners. This is in essence about providing the 'continuing support and development of all staff so that they possess the competencies, knowledge, skills and experience – necessary for the delivery of a safe, effective and patient-centred service' (DoH 2005, p. 7).

This involves identifying and dealing with acute and localised problems in care associated with skills deficit as well as facilitating long-term changes across the organisation. Applying a systematic approach, such as the one described here, is useful since it facilitates critical consideration of key issues in the process of sharing critical care skills.

While the underlying assumption is that education leads to changes in practice, the reality is that such change requires a pluralistic approach in order that the clinical, individual, system and organisational changes required are supported by the appropriate policies, guidelines, resources and culture.

Five years on from *Comprehensive Critical Care* (DoH 2000) the findings of the NCEPOD (2005) report *An Acute Problem?* show that whatever the successes of critical care outreach there is still much to do.

REFERENCES

Audit Commission (1999) *Critical to Success: The Place of Efficient and Effective Critical Care Services within the Acute Hospital.* Oxford: Audit Commission Publications.

Bassey M (1999) *Case Study Research in Educational Settings*. Milton Keynes: Open University Press.

Benner P (1984) *From Novice to Expert: Excellence and Power in Clinical Nursing Practice*. Menlo Park, California: Addison-Wesley.

Benner P, Tanner CA, Chelsa CA (1996) *Expertise in Nursing Practice: Caring, Clinical Judgement and Ethics*. New York: Springer Publishing Co.

Brookfield SD (1986) *Understanding and Facilitating Adult Learning*. Milton Keynes: Open University Press.

Cervero RM (1985) Continuing professional education and behavioural change: a model for research and evaluation. *Journal of Continuing Education in Nursing* 16(3): 85–8.

Cioffi J (2000) Recognition of patients who require emergency assistance: a descriptive study. *Heart & Lung* 29: 262–8.

Coad S, Haines S (1999) Supporting staff caring for critically ill patients in acute care areas. *Nursing in Critical Care* 4(5): 245–8.

Covey S (1989) *The 7 Habits of Highly Effective People*. New York: Simon & Schuster.

Crighton IM, Winter RJ (1997) Failure to recognise the need for readmission to an intensive care or high dependency unit. *British Journal of Intensive Care* 7(2): 46–8.

Cutler LR (2000) Competence in context. *Nursing in Critical Care* 5(6): 294–9.

Cutler LR (2002) From ward-based critical care to educational curriculum 2: A focussed ethnographic case study. *Intensive and Critical Care Nursing* 18(4).

Daffurn K, Lee A, Hillman KM, Bishop GF, Bauman A (1994) Do nurses know when to summon emergency assistance? *Intensive and Critical Care Nursing* 10: 115–20.

Department of Health (2000) *Comprehensive Critical Care, A Review of Adult Critical Care Services*. London: The Stationery Office.

Department of Health (2001) *the Nursing Contribution to the Provision of Comprehensive Critical Care for Adults: A Strategic Programme of Action*. London: Department of Health.

Department of Health (2005) *Quality Critical Care: Beyond 'Comprehensive Critical Care'. A Report by the Stakeholder Forum*. London: Department of Health.

Ferrell MJ (1988) The relationship of continuing education offerings to self-reported change in behaviour. *Journal of Continuing Education in Nursing* 19: 21–4.

Francke AL, Garssen B, Abu-Saad G (1995) Determinants of changes in nurses' behaviour after continuing education: a literature review. *Journal of Advanced Nursing* 21(2): 371–7.

Gibson J (1998) Using the Delphi technique to identify the content and context of nurses continuing professional development needs. *Journal of Clinical Nursing* 7(5): 451–9.

Gorard D (1999) Suboptimal care should have been defined (Letter to the Editor). *British Medical Journal* 318: 51.

Grant J, Stanton F (1998) *The Effectiveness of Continuing Professional Development*. 2nd revised edition. London: Joint Centre for Education in Medicine.

Haines S, Coad S (2001) Supporting ward staff in acute care areas: expanding the service. *Intensive & Critical Care Nursing* 17(2): 105–9.

Heap M, Cockbill-Black S, Bond J (1999) An audit of 'at risk' patients within the Northern General Hospital NHS Trust. Unpublished.

Heick MA (1981) Continuing education impact evaluation. *Journal of Continuing Education in Nursing* 12(4): 15–23.

Intensive Care Society (2002) *Guidelines for the Introduction of Outreach Services.* London: Intensive Care Society.

Jordan S (1999) Assessing educational effectiveness: the impact of a specialist course on the delivery of care. *Journal of Advanced Nursing* 30(4): 796–807.

Jordan S (2000) Educational input and patient outcomes: Exploring the gap. *Journal of Advanced Nursing* 31(2): 461–71.

Jordan S, Hughes D (1998) Using bioscience knowledge in nursing: actions, interactions and reactions. *Journal of Advanced Nursing* 27(5): 1060–8.

McGloin H, Adam S, Singer M (1997) The quality of pre-ICU care influences outcomes of patients admitted from the ward. *Clinical Intensive Care* 8: 104.

McQuillan P, Pilkington S, Allan A, Taylor B, Short A, Morgan G et al. (1998) Confidential enquiry into quality of care before admission to intensive care. *British Medical Journal* 316: 1853–8.

Metcalf A, McPherson K (1995) *Study of the Provision of Intensive Care Provision in Intensive Care in England, 1993: Revised Report for the Department of Health.* London: London School of Hygiene and Tropical Medicine.

Modernisation Agency (2003) *The National Outreach Report 2003: Progress in Developing Services.* London: Department of Health and Modernisation Agency.

Murch P, Warren K (2001) Developing the role of critical care liaison nurse. *Nursing in Critical Care* 6(5): 221–5.

National Confidential Enquiry into Perioperative Deaths (1999) *Extremes of Age: The 1999 Report of the National Confidential Enquiry into Perioperative Deaths.* London: NCEPOD.

National Confidential Enquiry into Perioperative Deaths (2005) *An Acute Problem?* London: NCEPOD.

Neale G, Woloshynowych M, Vincent C (2001) Exploring the causes of adverse events in NHS hospital practice *J R Soc Med* 94(7): 322–30.

Oxman AD (1994) *No Magic Bullets.* London: North East Thames Regional Health Authority.

Roethlisberger FJ, Dickinson WJ (1939) *Management and the Worker.* Harvard, MA: Harvard University Press.

Rogers C (1969) *Freedom to Learn.* Columbus: Charles E Merrill.

Rogers EM, Shoemaker FF (1971) *Communication of Innovations.* New York: The Free Press.

Sheperd J (1995) Findings of a training needs analysis for qualified nurse practitioners. *Journal of Advanced Nursing* 22(1): 66–71.

Sotto E (1994) *When Teaching Becomes Learning.* London: Cassell.

Stein LI (1967) The doctor-nurse game. *Archives of General Psychiatry* 16: 699–703.

Wallis CB, Davies HTO, Shearer AJ (1997) Why do patients die on general wards after discharge from intensive care? *Anaesthesia* 52: 9–14.

5 Case study: the use of high level clinical simulation in critical care nurse education

LEE CUTLER AND JUDITH CUTLER

INTRODUCTION

This case study gives an overview of an innovation in critical care education – the RAMSI Course (Recognition and Management of the Seriously Ill). The course was developed and delivered at the Montagu Clinical Simulation Centre, part of Doncaster and Bassetlaw Hospitals NHS Foundation Trust. A summary of initial evaluation is presented as well as a summary of key issues for teachers and learners involved in this type of education.

THE NEED FOR A DIFFERENT KIND OF CRITICAL CARE EDUCATION

In the National Outreach Report of 2003 it was acknowledged that

> many staff have difficulty with the practicalities of managing acutely ill patients. Therefore, education must integrate appropriate theory with opportunities to practise key psychomotor skills, ideally with work in simulated or real clinical situations. In the future, clinical simulators may have a particularly useful role in such training. (Modernisation Agency 2003)

When *Comprehensive Critical Care* was published we were both working in clinical roles with an educational remit. We had both taught on many critical care education programmes. These ranged from university-based intensive-care nursing courses, skills centre-based trauma workshops within pre-registration curricula, hospital-based critical care theory and skills programmes as well as Resuscitation Council Advanced Life Support courses. In addition we had developed a clinical competency framework for level 1, 2 and 3 areas. We had worked with nurses at bedside and attempted to integrate theory and practice as far as possible. But as any practice-based educator knows those teaching moments when the student says 'ah ha – now I understand' come through hard work and opportunism. It is often that one has to wait for the right clinical experiences while trying to cram their learning into a tight schedule of your workload and their learning of the key things they 'need to know'. The integration of theory and practice is problematic and requires expert facilitation. When critical care skills are to be shared throughout the hospital, opportunistic clinical teaching is not sufficient and this cannot be sufficiently compensated for through classroom-based programmes.

Around this time a clinical simulation centre was commissioned and we were invited to contribute to the range of courses that would be delivered there. After spending some time playing with the mannequin and computers that control its physiology, it soon became apparent that this had unique educational potential (Box C5.1). One could almost bring any patient-related situation or clinical problem into a safe environment for learning.

We had tried simulation-based teaching in lots of guises but never felt that it was quite right. When the 'teacher' is present the 'learner' looks for approval. With limited technology the level of physiological/clinical data is poor. The 'teacher' speaking as the patient does little to help the learner stay focused on the mannequin rather than the 'teacher'. It is often the case that learners are asked to act in roles that are different from their usual clinical role. The result is that they focus so much on what they think professionals would do that it inhibits critical thinking and reflection on their own role and habits of thought and action.

CLINICAL SIMULATORS IN CLINICAL EDUCATION

High-fidelity simulators were first introduced for training aircraft pilots. The training included how to handle situations where things go wrong. The first simulators used for training medical personnel were invented in 1986 by a Stanford physician (Vandrey and Whitman 2001). Their early use was for training anaesthetists and this has continued since. There are several modern 'high-fidelity' simulators, or in other words 'advanced computer controlled simulators' in the UK. The UK simulators have generally been used by anaesthetists to teach them such skills as crisis avoidance and management, as well as anaesthetic techniques within a simulated theatre setting. More recently, in North America, simulators have been used to simulate environments in which acute and critical care skills can be taught to nurses (Vandrey and Whitman 2001). However, simulator-based teaching such as this is the exception in Europe (Figure C5.1).

Box C5.1 What the mannequin can do

- Blinks its eyes and can be altered to simulate different levels of consciousness or anxiety
- Pupils – normal size and reaction to light or react abnormally as programmed
- Breaths with symmetrical/asymmetrical chest movement as programmed, generating normal breath sounds or a range of abnormal breath sounds
- Inhales/exhales normal O_2 and CO_2 levels and thus can be monitored with capnometry
- Has 'normal' airway anatomy that can occlude, be intubated with ET tube, tracheostomy etc.
- Has 'normal' lung physiology that can have CPAP and non-invasive ventilation via face mask or be mechanically ventilated and react to the ventilation in various ways as prescribed (e.g. bronchospasm, reduced compliance)
- Can have a chest drain inserted and needle decompression for pneumothorax
- 'Talks' via a speaker in the mannequin's throat linked to a microphone in the control room
- Has palpable peripheral and central pulses
- Can be cannulated and given IV fluid
- When catheterised passes 'urine' in response to administered fluid and blood pressure
- Generates normal heart sounds, additional sounds and murmurs as programmed
- When connected to a bedside monitor generates invasive BP, CVP, PAP, ECG, SPO_2
- Reacts physiologically to any drug that is used in the management of the seriously ill (e.g. inotropes, sedatives, muscle relaxants, bronchodilators)

THE RAMSI COURSE

The course was developed and delivered by nurses for nurses in order to meet the contemporary educational demands for developing and enhancing the critical care skills of staff in the acute wards. The aims of the course were:

- to facilitate the development of competence in the recognition and care of acutely critically ill patients;

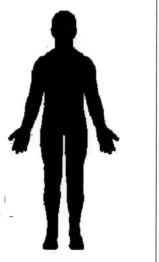

Clinical room

Setup as a fully equipped clinical area (e.g. ICU, Surgical ward, A&E)

Monitoring and technical equipment displays and reacts to the physiology of the mannequin (e.g. BP, ECG, CVP, PAP, SpO$_2$, ventilator readings, ETCO$_2$)

A healthcare technician accompanies the students who are in the 'hot seat', helping them to use equipment and receiving instructions from the control room team

Control room

One-way mirror and video link to clinical room

From here all physiological parameters can be monitored and altered via central computer system linked to the mannequin

The scenario facilitators observe, control and act as the voice of the patient (via a microphone to a speaker in the mannequin) and those contacted by telephone from the clinical room (e.g. doctors on-call, switchboard)

From here the clinical room activity is video taped for play back during debrief at the end of the scenario

Observation/debrief room

One-way mirror / video link to clinical room

From here all physiological parameters are displayed on a slave monitor

Those students not in the 'hot seat' for the scenario observe their fellow students as the scenario unfolds

Following the scenario all students watch the video of the scenario and there is a group debrief

Figure C5.1 Inside the simulator suite.

- to respond to the imperatives facing current and future practitioners within acute/critical care environments;
- to provide a learning environment that effectively facilitates learning and actively supports and promotes a holistic approach to the care of the acutely critically ill.

In meeting these aims explicit learning outcomes were articulated as a basis for developing the course and focusing the activity of the learners and teachers. The course learning outcomes were focused on the following areas:

- a thorough and systematic approach to the assessment of the critically ill patient and the overall clinical situation, paying appropriate attention to relevant detail;
- appropriate and timely intervention according to the practitioner's level and scope of practice;
- summoning appropriate help and making a concise but comprehensive presentation of the important issues relevant to the care and needs of the patient;
- effective leadership and/or follower skills that are appropriate to the situation and the practitioner's professional role and level of practice;
- anticipation of problems/potential problems and action to prevent or proactively manage them;
- effective communication within complex clinical situations;
- appropriate professional attitude and behaviour expected of a fully integrated member of the multi-disciplinary healthcare team;
- sound evaluative judgements and justification of these based on the clinical needs of the patient.

The course is delivered over a single day. The day is introduced with ice-breaking and discussion of what the day involves. There is a brief seminar focusing on systematic patient assessment, situation assessment and team leadership and follower skills. The remainder of the day comprises four clinical scenarios and debriefing after each one where the whole group of those attending the course view the video recording of the scenario. Each scenario lasts between 10 and 25 minutes depending on how the team deal with the problems it presents. Each debrief lasts between 30 and 45 minutes depending on what issues are raised in the scenario and debrief.

The scenarios are drawn from a database that we have built up over the years. They are all taken from real life events and cover problems including reduced level of consciousness, circulatory shock, respiratory failure and renal dysfunction, in isolation or combination. Additional problems include anaphylaxis and medical equipment failures. The information available for the team includes: case notes, prescription sheet, clinical observation charts and fluid balance charts, chest X-rays, 12-lead ECG and blood results, as well as repetition of any further tests such as arterial blood gases following intervention. As the scenario progresses the nurses maintain notes and observation charts as they would in real life. They are in the clinical room as a team alone. Any help they call for is via a telephone which is connected to the control room where switchboard, the on-call doctors and laboratories, for example, can be contacted and consulted. The facilitators act as family/visitors and medical staff who attend within a reasonable time if they are convinced they should, given their current workload or priorities in other departments! The scenarios are specifically selected for each group in order that the history and initial brief to the group is appropriate to their clinical area.

The debrief is extremely important. One of the course facilitators is allocated to debrief each scenario. From the commencement of the scenario their single role is to watch the events and take notes. They note the times at which key events occur and when interesting issues are raised in the scenario. This is then used to punctuate the debrief by way of fast forwarding the video to key events. Debrief is discussed in greater depth below.

INITIAL EVALUATION

The course was delivered as a pilot over a year. Below are details from the evaluation of the first nine RAMSI courses delivered in 2003/04. It comprises responses to statements about the RAMSI course based on a Likert scale (Table C5.1) as well as a sample of the anonymous free-text comments that learners made. Details of the grades of staff who attended the course are also presented in Table C5.2.

A selection of the anonymous free text comments made by the learners included the following.

Worth every bit of anxiety. Thanks.
An excellent learning experience.
Although daunting at first, it ended up being a valuable day's training with positive outcomes.
Really enjoyable day – constructive to work with others as makes you evaluate your own practice. Made a big difference wearing uniforms – made you feel more in 'work mode' than previous study days and enjoyed working with work colleagues/friends.
Very relaxed atmosphere and the course helped to make it less intimidating and positive feedback to all groups was good.
I found the course informative and enjoyable, the video feedback was interesting.
Very effective teaching method – excellent with feedback. Friendly staff – very constructive, really enjoyed it.
Good idea to attend with colleagues whom you regularly work with.

SALIENT ISSUES

There are innumerable issues that are worthy of discussion here and that the reader interested in education may find relevant. However, in this brief case study there is scope to share just a few of these issues, in particular the lessons we learned.

While we have referred to 'teachers' in this case study they are not teachers in the traditional sense. It is more accurate to refer to them as facilitators in the context of simulation. Their role is to support, facilitate and challenge the learners as they work through scenarios. In doing this they observe their own

Table C5.1 Evaluation summary

Statement	Strongly agree	Tend to agree	Uncertain	Tend to disagree	Strongly disagree
The course was enjoyable	74	7	1		
The course was relevant to my work	76	10	1		
I found the scenarios challenging	72	12			
The debriefing was constructive	76	10	1		
I felt able to ask any questions	73	12	1		
I feel better able to manage crises in the future	65	22	1		
This type of training will improve patient safety	66	13	1		
The length of the course was just right	63	9	1		
The course was well organised	81	3	1		
This type of training should be repeated every 1–2 years	72	12	2		
I found it easy to get time off to attend the course	66	15	1	2	
I would recommend the course to colleagues	81	4	1		

Table C5.2 Nurses attending the pilot courses

Job	Sister/charge nurse	Physio	Staff nurse	Nurse practitioner	HCSW
Number	23	3	51	2	7

performance on video and grapple with the reality of how they can learn from their acute awareness of how they really react and behave when faced with a situation which goes awry. This process is not always painless and as a facilitator one never knows what will happen next. Part of the expertise of facilitation is being comfortable with this and knowing what principles are guiding your role. We have heard ourselves say time and time again phrases such as 'It is not the purpose of the day to test or make judgements about your practice.' Rather we try to help individuals and teams identify and discuss the best way to act. Admitting one's own past mistakes and misunderstandings goes a long way to creating an atmosphere where imperfection is normal and where what matters is learning and moving on.

It is obvious from the evaluative comments we have included above that the learners did find the experience challenging – perhaps even intimidating, stressful and frightening. However, these appear to be balanced with comments referring to the fact that it was 'all worth it' and that they actually enjoyed it. In all our educational endeavours we pride ourselves on challenging learners in a relationship where we are very informal, we laugh with them, and also ensure that faults and failures are seen as priceless opportunities to give someone an increased sense of self-esteem and confidence through learning. Above all, learning is seen as the learners' responsibility: we are just there to make the process less painful and whenever possible point out the successes we see. Learners have to walk away from the day feeling positive and valued as well as challenged. This is why the skill of debrief is so important.

A major strength of simulation is that, unlike real life, time to debrief the situation is provided. The most powerful aspect of this is watching a video recording of the whole scenario as it occurred. Individuals are generally overly self-critical. This is where the messiness of real life and what it is realistic to expect of oneself is a common theme in our comments. As teachers it is always encouraging to see how much attention is paid to each part of the course. Learners put great effort into concentrating and discussing the issues inherent in each scenario and the actions of the team dealing with it. Box C5.2 includes a list of prompts we draw from to facilitate the debrief.

Box C5.2 Structured debrief

Debrief

- *Address to team/observers*
  'How did that go?' (keep brief but allow to calm down and address immediate anxieties)
  'What went well?' (focus on positives and points for improvement will be dealt with during the course of the debrief – don't allow to side track – aim to keep debrief in sequence according to the scenario)
- *Show relevant clips from video – as noted by 'debriefer'*
  'What were you thinking at this point?'
  'What did you think was going on at this point?'
  'Tell us about what you were doing at this point'
  'How could you have done that differently?'
  'What other actions/approaches might have helped here?'
  'How did you feel at this point / when x said . . . / when x happened?'
- *FF past low activity periods/periods not of interest*

Debrief of individual and interpersonal behaviour (probes/questions)

- Did the nominated leader act like a leader?
- Did the leader have a significant presence in the room?
- What was the leader and team members' position in the room/proximity to the patient?
- Did the leader deal well with unexpected events?
- Were events declared?
- Were goals of behaviour/approach/interventions stated/re-stated?
- Did the leader deal well with any dissent or other challenging team behaviour?
- Was the leader at the centre of communication channels?
- Was verbal communication within the team clear and unambiguous?
- What does the non-verbal communication of the leader and team members indicate?
- Was delegation appropriate?
- Did followers continuously feed back to leader?
- Did the followers accept delegated responsibility?
- Did the followers offer appropriate technical and psychological support?

* Did the leader repeatedly review the situation?
* How was the overall teamwork?

Closure of debrief

* Invite questions
* Offer summary and leave with positive comments ('criticism sandwich')

Earlier we referred to our belief that having established teams take part in the course was beneficial. On the RAMSI course we tried to ensure that this determined who attended. However, there were occasions when individuals worked in teams with those they would not usually work with. One case was where the outreach teams from our clinical network attended the course. This highlighted dynamics in relationships that would not be evident in any other mode of teaching. This presented challenges for the course facilitators and reinforced our belief that simulation, on this level, deals with difficult and complex aspects of practice that are not usually dealt with through education and that are important determinants of team effectiveness in practice and in crisis. Established teams present the greatest potential for allowing learners to observe, reflect on and learn from their performance. Otherwise they are often distracted by the fact that things aren't as they would usually be within the team.

Because the scenarios were from real life, and because the teams were real teams, real issues from practice emerged and had to be dealt with. One issue that was a recurrent theme in every course was that of role boundaries, including adding to or subtracting from medical orders. In particular commencing and titrating oxygen and fluids was a particularly frequent issue. This has prompted us to take these issues back to practice and support our nursing colleagues on acute wards with patient group directions for oxygen and IV fluid administration and titration.

The list of what the mannequin can do may conjure an image of a near human model, especially to those who have not seen the model in real life. However, it does have limitations and learners soon realise these when they are exposed to a simulated scenario. The nuances of skin colour and moisture, as well as facial expression and non-verbal signals, are extremely significant qualitative cues used by clinicians to assess patients in practice. These cannot be simulated and this leaves the simulation student relying mainly on 'hard' clinical data. The only break from this is the patient's voice and verbal cues that the patient is confused, agitated, breathless, in pain or suddenly less responsive than a few minutes earlier, for example. This requires some amateur dramatic skills from the course facilitators.

No matter what the technological advances of the future the interaction of the expert teacher and learner remains central to learning for practice.

THE FUTURE

Following a successful pilot of the RAMSI course there are plans to continue the programme building it into the mandatory training of junior medical staff and into the range of critical care education offered to acute ward nurses. Having piloted the course, we are now able to articulate the benefits and learning potential for *any* member of a clinical team; the course will in future be truly multi-disciplinary. This builds on and develops themes that were seen in the ALERT course but takes the simulation to a much more advanced level. Furthermore the learning comes through experience, critical reflection and structured debrief rather than theory-based principles or dogma.

While some evaluation of high-level simulation has been undertaken, showing positive results (Weller et al. 2003) further research and evaluative work are required before its benefits and limitations can be fully appreciated.

This novel approach to facilitating critical care skills and knowledge development seems to have great potential but is highly demanding on resources and the national picture of simulation is currently one of limited provision. Future work and investment in simulation are required.

REFERENCES

Modernisation Agency (2003) *The National Outreach Report 2003: Progress in Developing Services*. London: Department of Health and Modernisation Agency.

Vandrey C, Whitman K (2001) Simulator training for novice critical care nurses: preparing providers to work with critically ill patients. *American Journal of Nursing* 101(9): 24GG–24LL.

Weller J, Wilson L, Robinson B (2003) Survey of change in practice following simulation-based training in crisis management. *Anaesthesia* 58: 471–9.

6 Role expansion and the critical care outreach nurse

LEE CUTLER AND DENISE HONNOR

INTRODUCTION

The key aims of this chapter are briefly to explore some of the background and historical context of role expansion, to consider the issues surrounding role expansion for outreach practitioners specifically and finally to discuss some of the principles and practicalities of role expansion. A special area also considered in the chapter is that of nurse prescribing since this is the most significant area of role expansion in contemporary nursing. This chapter is followed by a case study that presents an example of role expansion that was undertaken in order to address the problems faced by nurses in one outreach team around the commencement and titration of oxygen. The chapter, and subsequent case study, will be of interest to nurses and allied health professionals working in critical care outreach.

HISTORICAL CONTEXT OF ROLE EXPANSION

Nurses taking on new roles and pursuing new areas of practice have a long history. Nursing is dynamic and ever-changing. The Briggs report (Briggs 1972) is one of the first artefacts from the fairly recent past which advocated that nurses should take on such tasks, usually of a medico-technical nature, that have traditionally been associated with the role of doctors. Subsequently guidelines were issued by the Department of Health and Social Security (DHSS 1977) which considered the legal and ethical implications of 'extended roles'.

A feature of 'extended' roles was an ethos of permission granted by medical staff and validated by certificates. Protocols and guidelines were issued and nurses undertaking expanded roles remained 'dependent' on medical staff.

As nursing evolved into the 1990s significant professional changes were seen. The professional maturation of nursing was acknowledged in Department of Health strategy (DoH 1993) and in professional literature of the time

Critical Care Outreach. Edited by Lee Cutler and Wayne Robson.
Copyright 2006 by John Wiley & Sons Ltd.

(Salvage 1992). In line with this change the United Kingdom Central Council for Nurses published *The Scope of Professional Practice* (UKCC 1992). The document was widely regarded as having moved nursing practice from its previous reliance on certification for tasks, towards an acceptance that it should be limited only by the individual accountable practitioner's own knowledge and competence (UKCC 2000).

Role 'expansion' is based on an alternative set of values to those associated with 'extended roles'. The values are about movement towards a more personal, effective and holistic practice (Wright 1995). It is also argued that expanded practice involves clinical decision-making and has education and skill as a basis (Maguire 1980). It is the acquisition of the necessary skill and underpinning knowledge and judgement that develops the nurse beyond basic training rather than the performance of tasks.

More recently further changes in nursing and allied health professions have involved increased autonomy and acknowledgement of advanced levels of practice. Traditional role boundaries and medical paternalism are increasingly being replaced by individual competence and patient need as determinants of nursing roles and scope of practice. Furthermore, career progression and financial rewards are more closely linked to what people actually do rather than what they know through the government's human resource strategy *Agenda for Change* (DoH 1999a).

One of the most significant examples of increased autonomy and the extent to which nurses are expanding their roles in contemporary nursing is the prescribing of medicines, which will be discussed in greater detail later in the chapter. Nurse prescribing differs significantly from many other areas of role expansion and may not be thought of in the same way as traditional tasks associated with 'scope'. It requires significant diagnostic and therapeutic judgement and knowledge and more representatively exemplifies expanded nursing practice than does venepuncture or other technical tasks, for example. It is therapeutic and holistic in its goals and aims to expedite timely treatment and alleviate suffering.

It could be argued that in recent years nurses have been liberated and empowered to achieve their potential in contributing in a wide range of areas associated with problems in health and well-being. This is evident from the plethora of services which are nurse-led, and from the ways in which patients are benefiting from the expert knowledge and skill which exists within the nursing profession and on which modern health services now depend. Critical care outreach is an example of one such service.

The approach to role expansion adopted by the nursing profession, first expounded in the *Scope of Professional Practice* (UKCC 1992), recognises that every nurse is accountable for their practice and that it is their professional judgement that can provide innovative solutions to meeting the needs of patients and clients in a modern dynamic health service. In their evaluation of *Scope* the UKCC stated:

This is a revolutionary approach. It means that new services can be set up with nurses, midwives and health visitors themselves deciding what skills and knowledge they need, without having to collect certificates task by task. It puts the onus on the individual practitioner to define the limits of their practice and to refer to appropriate others when necessary. (UKCC 1997)

This statement suggests that individual competence is the only factor limiting practice. However, it is important to acknowledge the reality in relation to limits on practice. In fact the organisation that a nurse works for (e.g. the hospital) will inevitably place limits on his or her practice through vicarious liability. Vicarious liability is simply where the organisation a nurse works for assumes liability for their actions so long as they are working within agreed organisational boundaries and to agreed standards. Thus, in reality role expansion is usually about local practices which address the healthcare needs of patients undergoing assessment and receiving care in specific clinical services.

ROLE EXPANSION IN THE CONTEXT OF CRITICAL CARE OUTREACH

Very little discussion of role expansion by critical care outreach nurses has been seen in the literature. One notable exception is the *National Outreach Report* (Modernisation Agency 2003) which acknowledged that among the key skills for outreach nurses are venepuncture and cannulation. Examples of oxygen and fluid administration through patient group directions were also cited in the report.

Within the broader context of critical care nursing, role expansion is generally accepted as a part of everyday practice. However, the influence of local context and culture on practice among professional groups is significant. This has resulted in a rich diversity in the range and type of expanded roles undertaken by critical care nurses nationally as well as internationally. Quite simply what is seen to be acceptable by one group in one organisation may not be acceptable in another context. Thus it is not surprising that when critical care nurses begin to practise outside of the familiar ICU or HDU community a phase of re-assessment of role expansion is deemed necessary. In our experience nurses describe a feeling of initial insecurity and uncertainty about the boundaries of practice and role as well as the level of support they perceive.

Outreach poses special challenges for the critical care nurse. The level of experience, professional judgement and maturity needed to work through the issues related to role boundaries and expansion is considerable. One of the challenges is a result of the nature of critical illness as it occurs in the general ward – outside of the secure, well-resourced, environment of critical care.

Often at this phase of critical illness patients are unstable and present with a range of very complex and inter-related clinical problems. A focused and directed assessment is required followed by rapid life-preserving interventions such as airway maintenance, oxygen therapy or fluid resuscitation. Evidence and international consensus both indicate that rapid assessment and early goal directed intervention improve survival in the critically ill. The case of severe sepsis serves as one salient example which has received significant attention recently (Rivers et al. 2001; Dellinger et al. 2004).

For some time 'Identifying and managing a patient crisis until physician assistance is available' (Benner 1984) has been acknowledged as an important and legitimate function of the nurse. It is one which requires considerable knowledge, skill and a high level of clinical judgement. Situations where patients are in life-threatening deterioration are part of the daily work of outreach nurses. When medical staff are not present nurses are required to walk a fine line between not jeopardising the patient's life by withholding necessary life support measures and at the same time working within the bounds of safe nursing practice (Benner 1984).

Where local policies do not exist to support and guide the nurse in this element of the role this omission only serves to perpetuate the dilemma that nurses face when doctors are absent and patients require intervention. The use of patient group directions, for example, can give nurses the legitimate authority as well as the professional and legal 'protection' necessary.

Outreach nursing, however, is not just about acting in the absence of medical staff. Many situations arise where despite medical presence advanced judgement and intervention through expanded roles are required of the nurse. This has been referred to as 'experiential leadership' (Benner et al. 1999, p. 211) and is important when the legitimate leader is inexperienced or is unable to provide appropriate or adequate medical direction or skilled know-how. In this situation the experienced nurse may feel morally compelled to take the lead in managing or coaching the management of the patient to ensure safe, timely and appropriate care (Benner et al. 1999).

The need for outreach nurses to coach and lead junior doctors will probably always be a reality of practice. Despite several years of critical care outreach and a refocusing of hospital-based medical training to include recognition of the critically ill and the immediate management of fluid and oxygen therapy in these patients, audit of practice continues to identify care which is less than optimal (National Confidential Enquiry into Perioperative Deaths 2005). The wealth of experience that senior outreach nurses possess brings with it the ability to achieve a rapid clinical grasp of the situation and a knowledge of what needs to be done. This cannot be taught in medical school but the situation has probably been made worse by the inadequacies of current medical undergraduate education (Goldacre et al. 2003).

There is considerable potential for outreach nurses to demonstrate, lead and coach in areas that might be considered expanded roles. These areas are part of a holistic approach to the identification and management of the critically ill. Outreach nurses are well placed to know what needs to be done next as well as the principles and evidence base supporting early assessment and intervention. However, dilemmas clearly arise when nurses are not empowered to intervene or when the espoused model on which their outreach team is based advocates a 'hands-off' approach.

While a rich diversity of different models of outreach are seen in practice they appear to be situated somewhere on a continuum. At one extreme is a model which has existed in reality for many years, but which was probably first described by Coad and Haynes (1999). This advocates education as the way to improve the care of the critically ill proactively in the acute ward environment. At the other extreme of the continuum is the model where intervention by a 'medical emergency team' (Lee et al. 1995) advocates a rapid, reactive and interventionist response when someone is identified as being 'at risk'. As yet no one clear model has emerged as the 'best way' and in reality probably a balance is needed between education and intervention.

We have heard much debate that suggests some nurses are reluctant to intervene as this contradicts the educational model of practice they espouse. However, without pursuing a lengthy critique of the different models of outreach it is important to offer a perspective that outlines a third way – one where education and intervention are possible.

Intervening does not always mean taking over from the ward staff. It can mean demonstrating and role modelling what to do – this shows, by way of example, when, where and how to intervene. Role modelling is an extremely powerful way of teaching others in practice-based areas (Charters 1999). Conversely advice without a willingness to share tasks and engage in the often complex process of stabilisation may seem to have a hollow tone or may be perceived as lacking credibility. ('Do as I say not as I do.')

What matters is a philosophy which empowers and facilitates learning in practice. Such a philosophy and principles should be relied upon to guide what is most appropriate in any given situation and will not drive the practitioner to extreme models of practice where a monopoly on intervention or total abstinence results in outreach being perceived as a confused addition to existing clinical teamwork. Box 6.1 provides an example from practice.

PRINCIPLES AND PRACTICAL CONSIDERATIONS

It is important that practitioners who choose to expand their role have a comprehensive understanding of the key principles surrounding role expansion and are able to think critically about the application of these principles when making decisions about expanding their role. To this end it is considered useful to discuss some of the principles and practical considerations here.

Box 6.1 Case study: Doncaster and Bassetlaw critical care outreach team

While an overall philosophy guiding the team is one of empowerment, education and support, the reality remains that two factors influenced decisions about role expansion:

1. That supporting change and best practice in the care of the critically ill involves a willingness to stand beside the acute ward practitioner, of whatever discipline, and work with them demonstrating, teaching, supervising and advising on best care.
2. At times outreach nurses will be with patients who are in life-threatening decline and medical staff are not present and are delayed in attending.

For these reasons we planned to draw on existing professional and local policies to support role expansion in certain key areas. These were identified through audit of outreach work and clinical supervision with nurses working in the team. The key areas identified were:

Requesting pathology tests (e.g. U&Es, FBC, PG, ABG, LFT, clotting, blood cultures)
Requesting chest X-rays
Venepuncture
Peripheral venous cannulation
Arterial blood sampling by arterial puncture
Commencement and titration of oxygen (by PGD)
Administration of IV fluid bolus (by PGD)
Changing a tracheostomy and decannulation.

These are regularly undertaken by the nurses on the outreach team and have facilitated more timely care many instances. They have also built some common ground between junior medical staff and the outreach nurses.

The key principles of *The Scope of Professional Practice* (UKCC 1992), more recently incorporated into the *Code of Professional Conduct* (NMC 2002), are that nurses should:

• uphold the interests of patients and clients at all times;
• keep their knowledge, skills and competence up to date;

- recognise the limits of their own knowledge and skill and take appropriate action to address any deficiencies;
- ensure that existing standards of care are not compromised by new developments and responsibilities;
- acknowledge their own professional accountability for all actions and omissions;
- avoid inappropriate delegation.

The process of decision-making about role expansion is complex and should involve thorough consideration of the broad professional and legal principles as well as local clinical issues. The gravity of the situation and responsibility nurses take on when making decisions and intervening with critically ill patients cannot be overstated. The reality is that nurses face severe consequences if they fail to uphold good standards of care. Among these consequences are:

- prosecution by the state under criminal law;
- civil law action for damages;
- being struck off the professional register following a professional conduct hearing;
- disciplinary procedures or dismissal by employer.

The accountability and duty of care that outreach nurses have means that care will be judged according to professional and legal principles. Action or omission within one's duty of care will be judged against reasonable standards of practice in the circumstances. It is imperative that nurses strive to ensure they are competent in the roles they undertake. When these roles were previously undertaken by medical staff – this will provide the standard against which practice will judged (the Bolam principle).

As with all care it is important that consent is sought from the patient unless they are deemed incompetent. It is not unusual for critically ill patients to have altered consciousness; however, assumptions should not be made about the patient's ability to give consent. The NMC (2002) guidance suggests that 'every patient and client is legally competent unless otherwise assessed by a suitably qualified practitioner'. Furthermore the nurse can only act without consent for the preservation of life in extreme circumstances (NMC 2002).

Where difficulties arise and situations seem indeterminate then the local ethics forum and/or clinical governance committee should be consulted. Following the guidance provided by these bodies will ensure that vicarious liability is upheld and that the nurse is protected in her role. Additional sources of professional advice are the Nursing and Midwifery Council and unions such as the Royal College of Nursing which may be able to give a broader perspective based on examples from other organisations.

In essence protection is achieved through ensuring competence, and action only within one's sphere of competence, adherence to local policy, as well as through consent by the patient (unless acting to preserve life). Incorporating these into particular new areas of practice is not always as simple as it has been made to sound here. Good mentorship and clinical supervision are essential.

Now turning to more practical considerations, the reader is encouraged to reflect on the way role expansion may work within clinical services. Role 'expansion' and the *Scope of Professional Practice* (UKCC 1992) have changed the way nurses view their work. It has opened up more flexible and professionally challenging ways of developing practice. The experience and professional judgement of nurses can provide innovative solutions to meet the needs of patients (UKCC 1997). Critical care outreach nurses are in a key position to make decisions about how expansion of their role can improve clinical services for the critically ill. The following questions have been generated from the six principles of 'scope'. However, they also relate to clinical systems of care delivery as the context in which role expansion is considered. The questions are presented here as a framework to prompt reflection, critical thinking and help with planning for role expansion.

THE CURRENT SYSTEM OF CLINICAL CARE DELIVERY

Can you identify situations where care is less than optimal as a result of delay in, or inadequate performance of a particular task?

If you can answer 'yes' to this question this may be a situation where role expansion can improve the care for seriously ill patients, however, think also about the following.

- Is this role already the responsibility of one or more clinical professionals?
- Are these individuals aware that they have a responsibility for this role?
- Is the problem because of inadequate presence of health professionals?
- Are others unable to undertake the role because of other demands on their time? If so do systems need to be changed to allow their presence, or do seniors/managers need to be involved in ensuring that work and personnel are allocated more appropriately.
- Is the problem because of lack of skill, knowledge or experience on the part of those who are present with the patient?
- Is the problem because the particular role is not seen as useful within the culture or context of the local clinical environment?
- Do other things need to be done (education, audit, awareness raising, system redesign) instead of or as well as your role expansion?

YOUR POTENTIAL IMPACT ON THE SYSTEM

Will your role expansion optimise patient care and critical illness management?

- Will your role expansion help support system failures, even if you do not intend to build this into the service as a formal arrangement to be relied upon at all hours of the day?
- How will your role expansion work in the context of others who may be providing the same skills/role?
- Will other practitioners benefit from the teaching and support you will be able to offer?
- As well as undertaking the role in simple/uncomplicated situations, will you also be able to troubleshoot and help others less experienced than yourself (e.g. acute care nurses and medical staff in training)?
- Will your performance of the role reduce the opportunities for others to learn or enhance the opportunities for others to learn under your instruction and guidance?
- Will role expansion potentially impact significantly on your time – and if so can you manage this to ensure that your role is not diminished in other areas?
- Are there potential complications that may occur as a result of your role expansion? If so, how will you deal with these or ensure that systems are in place for others to deal with these if they should occur?
- What are the issues around consent for this type of role expansion?

YOUR PRACTICE AND DEVELOPMENT

What are the issues in developing and maintaining your competence?

- Is the role you wish to undertake already performed by other nurses in your organisation or will it be necessary to develop a proposal and learning/assessment package?
- How will you develop the skills and knowledge needed to perform the expanded role?
- Will you need a mentor? If so who can undertake this role?
- How will you ensure that you are competent?
- Will you perform the role frequently enough to ensure that your competence is maintained?

NURSE PRESCRIBING

The prescribing of medicines has been one of the most significant changes in the role of the nurse. The significance of the change is the reason why it has been included as part of this chapter since it stands as a special topic related to the expansion of the role of the nurse.

The changes necessary to allow this role expansion have included changes in law and professional policy. The Cumberledge Report (DHSS 1986) was the first official report to call for changes that would allow nurses to prescribe. In 1989 the Crown Report (DoH 1989) recommended that suitably qualified nurses (district nurses and health visitors) should be able to prescribe from the *Nurse Prescriber's Formulary (NPF)*.

Primary legislation was passed in 1992 and pilots for nurse prescribing occurred between 1994 and 1998. National roll-out of nurse prescribing was completed by 2001. At that time the formulary was very limited and still only allowed district nurses and health visitors to prescribe. However, the second Crown Report (DoH 1999b) recommended that prescribing be extended to other groups of nurses and non-medical professionals. This recommendation was then supported in the NHS Plan (DoH 2000a) and a government announcement to implement this came in 2001.

Subsequent changes have seen the introduction of supplementary prescribing and an increase in the range of medical conditions that can be treated, an increase in the *NPF* and that all GSL (general sales list) and pharmacy items can now be prescribed by nurse prescribers. The scope of non-medical prescribing is ever-increasing and offers tremendous potential for nurses to contribute their expertise in the care and treatment of patients. This includes those who are acutely and critically ill.

Currently, becoming a nurse prescriber requires completion of an academic programme of 25 taught days and 12 days in practice. The course is general in its content and is structured around general principles of prescribing rather than prescribing in a specific clinical speciality. Clearly a significant specialist knowledge base is needed in addition to the general principles of prescribing.

The competencies that support prescribing practice have been outlined by the National Prescribing Centre (2001) and are presented in Table 6.1. They

Table 6.1 Competencies that support prescribing practice

Competency area	Competencies
The consultation	Clinical and pharmacological knowledge Establishing options Communicating with patients
Prescribing effectively	Prescribing safely Prescribing professionally Improving prescribing practice
Prescribing safely	Information in context The NHS in context The team and individual context

include three areas of competence each with three specific competencies related to them.

These competencies are intended to ensure that the practice of those prescribing is safe and is underpinned by appropriate skill and knowledge. The principles outlined in the code of professional conduct (NMC 2002) also apply since they are broad enough to guide nurses in all areas of practice whether at the level of the newly registered nurse or at an advanced level of practice.

As well as a sound base of knowledge and experience in critical care nurse prescribing requires substantial additional training and ongoing development. This is in order to meet the legal and professional standards required which serve to ensure that good standards of practice are maintained. It could be argued that the resource costs of training and supporting nurses in prescribing are only justified if the conditions that the nurse can treat and the medicines they can prescribe are central to their speciality and role.

Our own internal audit has identified that the framework for nurse prescribing has expanded to a level where it includes many of the clinical problems that result in referral to critical care outreach. Common examples include:

- hypoxaemia (conditions requiring oxygen)
- exacerbations of asthma and COPD
- acute pulmonary oedema associated with cardiac failure
- hypovolaemia
- opioid overdose
- benzodiazepine overdose
- pain
- hypoglycaemia
- generalised tonic-clonic seizures.

Hence there is a great potential to impact upon the patient's condition which may be acutely life-threatening. The most recent change in nurse prescribing is the opening up of the whole *British National Formulary* from which nurses can prescribe within the limits of their competence. This offers great potential to improve patients' access to critical care.

If evidence exists locally that outreach can impact upon sub-optimal care through prescribing medicines – prescribing may be desirable. However, while treating these conditions is not beyond the scope of the nurse's practice it may be beyond the aims and scope of the outreach service. It may also meet with some objection from consultant medical staff or other members of parent teams. In this case the use of PGDs (patient group directions) may offer a solution since they can be developed by, or with the involvement of, physicians and surgeons, for example.

PGDs (previously called group protocols) were developed in response to the need for patients to receive medications administered to them by healthcare professionals without the need for an individual prescription from a prescriber. In 1998 the *Review of the Prescribing, Supply and Administration of Medicines* (DoH 1998) identified the benefits of group protocols, the law was clarified, and group protocols became known as *Patient Group Directions* following the issue of HSC 2000/26C in August 2000 (DoH 2000b). A PGD is described as:

> a written instruction for the sale, supply and/or administration of named medicines in an identified clinical situation. It applies to groups of patients who may not be individually identified before presenting for treatment. (DoH 2000b)

PGDs are subject to local interpretation which has allowed them to be used creatively in a wide range of circumstances. However, the guidance is that:

> the majority of clinical care should be provided on an individual basis. The supply and administration of medicines under PGD's should be reserved for those limited situations where this offers an advantage for patient care without compromising patient safety, and where it is consistent with appropriate professional relationships and accountability. (DoH 2000b)

PGDs have the additional benefit of not just allowing a few nurses to act – but for a much wider range of nurses/practitioners to administer drugs in acute life-threatening situations. We have pursued both models at Doncaster and Bassetlaw. Some members of the team prescribe while others act under PGDs. The conditions covered by PGDs include hypoxia and hypovolaemia and have resulted in a trust-wide framework that has also empowered appropriately trained acute ward nurses to intervene. One example, that of oxygen administration by PGD, is presented below by Elaine Shaw as a case study in role expansion.

In our experience there are many issues surrounding the development and use of PGDs – not to mention the potential for great difficulty surrounding a rational policy for fluid and oxygen administration for example. However, there are also great potential benefits. Our experience, though frustrating at times, required that a range of staff across the organisation engaged in constructive debate about ongoing contentious issues in the everyday practice of giving oxygen and IV fluids. Finding common ground is possible!

It is beyond the scope of this chapter to consider PGDs in any detail. However, detailed published guidelines are available and the reader is referred to them (see for example: National Prescribing Centre 2004; Royal Pharmaceutical Society of Great Britain 2004).

In summary the recent changes to the law and the introduction of a framework that supports the prescription of medicines, or the protocol guided administration of medicines without referral to a doctor using PGDs, are examples of 'role expansion' that have dramatically altered the boundaries of practice. A recent national evaluation of nurse prescribing concluded that nurses are prescribing frequently and clinically appropriately (Latter et al. 2005). The report found that the expansion of independent nurse prescribing is largely viewed as successful in a range of policy and practice dimensions. The benefits found included improving patients' access to medicines, utilising the expertise within nursing and reducing the dependence of nurses on medical staff to appropriately treat patients. The limitation of this study is that it was conducted at a time when nurse prescribing in acute and critical care was limited in relation to primary care, for example. Time, further research and future formulary expansion will allow a more valid evaluation of the impact of nurse prescribing in acute and critical care.

CONCLUSIONS

The role changes seen in contemporary nursing are based on an alternative set of values to those associated with the 'extended roles' of years ago. They emphasise movement towards more personal, effective and holistic practice. Features of contemporary expanded roles include clinical decision-making and autonomy based on appropriate experience, education and skill. This is exemplified in nurse prescribing where nurses can autonomously diagnose and treat medical conditions in order to relieve suffering and hasten recovery from illness. However, critical care is a challenging area for nurses to practise in this domain. Despite this there are other options open to nurses who wish to improve the access of critically ill patients to rapid treatment. Among these is the route of Patient Group Directions from which the nurse will gain greater support and shoulder less of the responsibility than with prescribing.

A set of principles, now incorporated into the code of conduct for nurses (NMC 2002), were outlined to guide nurses expanding their role. However, while role expansion is now at the core of many clinical services and nursing roles the case of critical care outreach is less than straightforward. Outreach services are often part-time, they may be primarily educative and supportive in their ethos and their team members are seen as 'visitors' on the wards. Because of these issues the questions outreach nurses are concerned with are not 'Can I expand my role?' rather they are 'Should I expand my role?' 'If I expand my role what if . . .?' and 'If I expand my role how will it impact and be perceived?'

It was not the aim of this chapter to answer these questions, rather to acknowledge their importance and set the debate outreach nurses may be having in context. A key challenge for outreach nurses in the future is to reason through the issues, and in the context of rapidly changing health services and nursing roles around them, decide how they can continue to make a unique contribution while adapting to meet patient needs.

REFERENCES

Benner P (1984) *From Novice to Expert: Excellence and Power in Clinical Nursing Practice.* Menlo Park, Calif.: Addison-Wesley.

Benner P, Hooper-Kyriakidis, Stannard D (1999) *Clinical Wisdom and Interventions in Critical Care: A Thinking in Action Approach.* Philadelphia: W B Saunders Co.

Briggs A (1972) *The Briggs Report. Report of the Committee on Nursing.* London: HMSO/DHSS.

Charters A (1999) Role modelling as a teaching method. *Emergency Nurse* 7(10): 25–9.

Coad S, Haines S (1999) Supporting staff caring for critically ill patients in acute care areas. *Nursing in Critical Care* 4(5): 245–8.

Dellinger RP, Carlet JM, Masur H et al. (2004) Surviving Sepsis Campaign guidelines for management of severe sepsis and septic shock. *Critical Care Medicine* 32(3): 858–73.

Department of Health (1989) *Report of the Advisory Group on Nurse Prescribing* (1st Crown Report). London: Department of Health.

Department of Health (1993) *A Vision for the Future.* London: Department of Health.

Department of Health (1998) *Review of Prescribing, Supply and Administration of Medicines: A Report on the Supply and Administration of Medicines under Group Protocols.* London: Department of Health.

Department of Health (1999a) *Agenda for Change: Modernising the NHS Pay System.* London: Department of Health.

Department of Health (1999b) *Review of the Prescribing, Supply, and Administration of Medicines* (2nd Crown Report). London: Department of Health.

Department of Health (2000a) *The NHS Plan.* London: Department of Health.

Department of Health (2000b) *Patient Group Directions* (England only) HSC 2000/26. London: Department of Health.

Department of Heath and Social Security (1977) *The Extended Role of the Clinical Nurse.* London: DHSS Circular HC(77) 22.

Department of Health and Social Security (1986) *Neighbourhood Nursing: A Focus for Care.* London: Cumberledge Report.

Goldacre M, Lambert T, Evan J, Turner G (2003) Preregistration house officers' views on whether their experience at medical school prepared them well for their jobs: national questionnaire survey. *British Medical Journal* 326(7397): 1011–12.

Latter S, Maben J, Myall M, Courtenay M, Young A, Dunn N (2005) *An Evaluation of Extended Formulary Independent Nurse Prescribing. Executive Summary of Final Report.* The University of Southampton, School of Nursing and Midwifery & Department of Health Policy Research Programme.

Lee A, Bishop G, Hillman K, Daffurm K (1995) The Medical Emergency Team. *Anaesthesia and Intensive Care* 23(2): 183–6.

Maguire JM (1980) *The Expanded Role of the Nurse.* London: King's Fund.

Modernisation Agency (2003) *The National Outreach Report 2003: Progress in Developing Services.* London: Department of Health and Modernisation Agency.

National Confidential Enquiry into Perioperative Deaths (2005) *An Acute Problem?* London: NCEPOD.

National Prescribing Centre (2001) *Maintaining Competency in Prescribing: An Outline Framework to Help Nurse Prescribers.* Liverpool: National Prescribing Centre.

National Prescribing Centre (2004) *Patient Group Directions: A Practical Guide and Framework of Competencies for all Professionals Using Patient Group Directions.* Liverpool: National Prescribing Centre.

Nursing and Midwifery Council (2002) *The NMC Code of Professional Conduct: Standards for Conduct, Performance and Ethics.* London: NMC.

Rivers E, Nguyen B, Havstad S et al. (2001) Early goal-directed therapy in the management of severe sepsis and septic shock. *New England Journal of Medicine* 345: 1368–77.

Royal Pharmaceutical Society of Great Britain (2004) *Patient Group Directions.* Fitness to Practise and Legal Affairs Directorate Fact Sheet: Ten. London: RPSGB.

Salvage J (1992) The new nursing: empowering patients or empowering nurses? In J Robson, A Gray, R Elkan (eds) *Policy Issues in Nursing.* Milton Keynes: Open University Press.

United Kingdom Central Council (1992) *The Scope of Professional Practice.* London: UKCC.

United Kingdom Central Council (1997) *Scope in Practice.* London: UKCC.

United Kingdom Central Council (2000) *Scope in Practice.* London: UKCC.

Wright S (1995) The role of the nurse: extended or expanded? *Nursing Standard* 9(33): 25–9.

6 Case study: expanding the role of the nurse in critical care outreach

ELAINE SHAW

INTRODUCTION

This case study outlines a project that aimed to address problems with administration and titration of oxygen therapy in the acutely/critically ill. In summary, patients were suffering because of system failures, dogma within and between professions and because of limitations on the scope of nursing practice. Many of the key issues that face outreach nurses considering role expansion are implicit in this case study. Much of the case study details appraisal of the problems since this is a key part of ensuring that the solution is holistic and does not simply result in additional tasks for the nurse to undertake. Through existing legal and professional frameworks the problems encountered were addressed. Part of the solution involved legitimising and supporting the role nurses have in administering and titrating oxygen therapy within collaborative respiratory therapy.

BACKGROUND

Awareness of the issues developed early on in the new role as an outreach nurse. The 'comfort zone' that nurses experience when working in intensive care units becomes apparent when it is lost. Before the change in role, the role boundaries and ability to work outside these with assumed consultant anaesthetic support were taken for granted. After working in the same ICU for many years the change to 'whole hospital cover', working with many unfamiliar staff, was unnerving.

Nurses in critical care regularly titrate life-supporting therapies and medication – even though this may not always be strictly within legal or professional frameworks. Acknowledged elements of expert nursing practice in critical care include assessing what can be safely added to or omitted from the medical prescription and how to manage life-threatening situations appro-

Critical Care Outreach. Edited by Lee Cutler and Wayne Robson.
Copyright 2006 by John Wiley & Sons Ltd.

priately in the absence of medical staff (Benner 1984; Benner et al. 1999). However, it is also acknowledged that changing the context of practice or entering a new speciality reduces the level at which professional practice and experts may suddenly feel like novices (Benner 1984). Thus the 'new' outreach nurse is confronted with an uncomfortable reality.

Situations regularly arose involving life-threatening physiological deterioration. Knowing what needed to be done was not an issue. However, feelings of insecurity and awareness of stepping outside the official boundaries significantly affected confidence, autonomy and fluency of practice. Furthermore, as an outreach nurse, leadership and role modelling best practice means considering how practice might be viewed or emulated by acute ward staff – so getting it right and having a clear policy is important.

During a clinical supervision session soon after joining the outreach service these issues and feelings were discussed with the consultant nurse for critical care. Oxygen administration was perceived as a significant problem. Conflicting advice from consultant medical staff, myths, dogma and failure to prescribe and monitor oxygen therapy were amongst the issues faced.

The problem was particularly relevant but complicated by the fact that Doncaster has the highest incidence of COPD (Chronic Obstructive Pulmonary Disease) in England (DoH 2002); a special problem for the critical care outreach team. Local physicians were understandably concerned that high-flow oxygen should not be given to all patients who presented with breathlessness. However, withholding oxygen in patients not at risk from high oxygen concentrations was also unsatisfactory.

The whole basis for nurses expanding their role is to ensure that care is holistic, timely and appropriate in order that patients benefit from nursing skill, knowledge and their constant bedside presence. The role expansion in this case needed to empower and guide nurses in timely and appropriate initiation and titration of oxygen therapy.

ISSUES WITH CLINICAL CARE

There were a number of issues and challenges which needed to be addressed by the nurses in the outreach team.

- Hypoxia is a life-threatening physiological problem that, in some instances, remains undetected and untreated.
- The adverse effects of oxygen in the few patients who suffer from hypoxic respiratory drive mean that there is no single dose of oxygen that could be considered safe for all. This has resulted in much dogma, conflict and mixed messages about how much oxygen to give. (NICE (2004) has acknowledged the adverse effects oxygen can have in some patients with COPD and advocated an upper limit for SpO_2 of 93%.)

- There is a general failure to set individualised targets for SaO_2, PaO_2 and $PaCO_2$ to guide administration and titration of oxygen therapy in the acutely ill.
- There is a general failure to prescribe oxygen in the way, and to the same standards, that other drugs are prescribed.
- Legally oxygen should be prescribed and so nurses are not at liberty to administer and titrate without protocols that are within current non-medical prescribing frameworks.
- Frequent failure to record how much oxygen is given (percentage of inspired O_2) in ward areas.
- Oxygen should be part of a treatment plan not a single measure to increase pulse oximetry readings.

OPTIONS FOR A SOLUTION

Some criteria were agreed in order to facilitate an appraisal of options. These were that the strategy must:

- be within legal and professional frameworks for nurses and physiotherapists;
- allow timely and autonomous administration and titration of oxygen;
- be part of holistic and comprehensive clinical guidelines for acute respiratory problems;
- be based on best evidence and expert opinion;
- be part of a strategy rather than just an additional task that nurses could 'do';
- have the potential to impact upon all acute areas where patients experience respiratory problems with minimal resource and training needs;
- improve the immediate care for patients experiencing acute respiratory problems.

A literature search was performed on the topics of oxygen prescribing and administration as well as a review of local practice. Consistent themes were poor practice around prescribing, administration and monitoring (Small et al. 1992; Dodd et al. 2000; Howell 2001). Lack of understanding and much disagreement among health professionals were also evident (Frazer and Crab 2002; O'Driscoll 2002; Thompson and Maxwell 2002). Some disease-specific guidelines were identified and it was considered that these could inform guidelines for acute care (e.g. BTS 2002; BTS and SIGN 2004; NICE 2004). In addition the legal and professional frameworks were studied to identify what scope and limitations surrounded prescribing or administering oxygen.

A range of options were considered but it was decided that to meet the set criteria a patient group direction (PGD) with an underpinning clinical algorithm was most appropriate. Patient group directions are written instructions for the administration of a named medicine in an identified clinical situation and apply to a group of patients who need not be individually identified before presenting for treatment (DoH, Health Service Circular 2000/026). This clearly allows non-medical professionals to administer (but not prescribe for others) oxygen.

Part of the appraisal of options included considering a set of questions that should be at the heart of any role expansion. Key responses to the questions are included here.

Does the patient benefit from nurses expanding their role in this way?

Yes, this will mean that nurses can intervene promptly when a life-threatening problem arises.

How will knowledge and skills be ensured and staff kept up-to-date?

Making key competencies explicit will allow training to be focused and ensure that staff undertaking the role will have a sound knowledge base for their practice.

How does it affect the nurse undertaking the role?

It will empower them, guide them and help them to work within a legal and professional framework guided by best evidence. It will not add to the nursing workload or take nurses away from other patients or duties since patient deterioration necessitates nursing presence in any case. However, the nurse will still be encouraged to call for medical help. The nurse will remain accountable for giving or withholding oxygen but hopefully the fear and dogma will be replaced with a rationale and evidence for action.

How does it affect other staff (e.g. doctors, nurses, physios)?

If the role expansion is taken up by many acute ward staff there are potentially widespread benefits. A systematic, logical and evidence-based approach to acute respiratory problems will allow practitioners to immediately intervene based on guidelines and competence not their professional background. However, guidance on when to call for medical or senior medical help will also ensure that the more seriously ill or those who do not respond to immediate and simple interventions will receive prompt expert/senior medical review and intervention building on initial assessment and intervention by other bedside staff.

How does it affect the system/outreach service?

If the role expansion is only for outreach nurses this may increase the dependence of ward staff on the team. However, if the role is taken up by a range of acute ward staff this will mean that the aims of the outreach team are being met without their direct intervention – though they would be available for support and guidance. This is particularly important as the outreach team intends to educate and empower ward staff and does not offer a 24-hour service.

DEVELOPING A PROTOCOL

Initial work was undertaken to identify the Trust framework for development of PGDs and explore how it had been used for other clinical problems and medication. However, it is fair to say that there is much which is unique about oxygen as a 'drug'. This meant that many of the usual questions and heading in the Trust's framework were difficult to answer or were irrelevant. The key challenge at this point was to keep assuring oneself that it was the framework which didn't quite fit the purpose rather than it being the project that was too difficult or unachievable. Perseverance ensured success in the end.

There was wide consultation and a small working group of key individuals. These included outreach nurses, a respiratory physician, an anaesthetist, and a physiotherapist. Process mapping identified key stages in the clinical process of patient assessment, commencement and titration of oxygen as well as other key interventions and considerations in evaluation and ongoing management. These were refined and discussed at length and were supported by evidence and expert opinion.

The final algorithm can be seen in Chapter 4 (see Figure 4.1) on 'Specific Clinical Problems'.

IMPLEMENTATION

The process of developing the PGD, the algorithm and group consensus and Trust approval was lengthy, taking 22 months in all.

The implementation was initially a pilot with intensive audit to ensure patient safety and identify any problem areas. The outreach nurses, senior physiotherapist and HDU sister were in the pilot group. All went well and the most difficult part was ensuring that staff completed the audit forms in order to evaluate the innovation.

Training, competence and assessment of competence were key issues for further 'roll-out'. Following the initial pilot, training involved two elements. First, the concept and use of PGDs was clarified. Secondly, the issues around safety, oxygen administration and acute respiratory problems were taught using case-based discussion workshops. The competencies required to undertake the role were documented in the PGD documentation, and the assessment of these competencies followed training sessions. The assessment involved an objective structured clinical examination (OSCE) and a viva (oral exam) where practitioners were invited to demonstrate and talk through the steps in patient assessment, oxygen therapy and collaboration with medical staff.

EVALUATION

There were no adverse incidents reported in the initial phase of use (or since). Significantly variables such as respiratory rate, SpO_2 and PaO_2 all improved with the algorithm use.

The audit also demonstrated that a whole range of interventions had been undertaken when patients became breathless. The commonest included changing patients' position, clearance of airway secretions, administration of bronchodilators, manoeuvres to manage the upper airway and the escalation of treatment to involve CPAP, NIV and admission to critical care for mechanical ventilation. Thus the PGD and the expanded role was not just being undertaken as a 'task' but, as intended, it was part of a comprehensive and collaborative approach to acute respiratory problems.

The PGD also allowed reduction of oxygen, and in many instances oxygen was reduced in recovering patients who had been on continuous oxygen for some time.

Lastly the core working group revised the algorithm based on experience and suggestions from other commentators in acute care. The changes included more clear distinctions between asthma and COPD, revised target levels for PaO_2 and SpO_2 in the COPD group and revision of phrasing for some points regarding ongoing evaluation and management.

THE FUTURE

The process of cascading the PGD for widespread use in acute clinical areas was commenced soon after initial pilot and evaluation. Key non-medical practitioners who care for patients with acute respiratory problems were targeted as those most likely to use the PGD. These included medical and surgical nurse practitioners, physiotherapists, registered nurses on acute medical and surgical wards, accident and emergency and perioperative areas.

The algorithm that forms the basis for the PGD is seen as a useful tool to help junior medical staff in their decisions and care. The clinical areas where the PGD is in use will display posters including the algorithm thus guiding multi-disciplinary care and facilitating anticipation and teamwork.

A further 'spin off' from the use of the PGD was yet another expanded role for outreach nurses – that of blood sampling via arterial puncture method. In the absence of medical staff this was seen to expedite rapid assessment and management.

REFLECTION ON LESSONS LEARNED

Changing whole systems is frustrating, challenging and takes time and perseverance. However, nurses are in a key position to bring about such change since they understand the implications of taking on new roles. Thus nurses should be at the centre of determining how expanded nursing roles should work in practice.

The process of changing and expanding nursing roles brings about significant learning and perspective transformation. In some instances, as with this case study, the role expansion involves legitimising and acknowledging the role nurses have in key elements of care. This supports the argument that individual professional groups no longer own roles or should be allowed to dictate care but that multi-disciplinary teams should work together to improve care.

REFERENCES

Benner P (1984) *From Novice to Expert: Excellence and Power in Clinical Nursing Practice.* Menlo Park, California: Addison-Wesley.

Benner P, Hooper-Kyriakidis P, Stannard D (1999) *Clinical Wisdom and Interventions in Critical Care: A Thinking-in-Action Approach.* Philadelphia: W B Saunders.

British Thoracic Society (2002) (British Thoracic Society Standards of Care Committee) Non-invasive ventilation in acute respiratory failure. *Thorax* 57: 192–211.

British Thoracic Society & Scottish Intercollegiate Guideline Network (2004) *British Guideline on the Management of Asthma* London: British Thoracic Society & Scottish Intercollegiate Guidelines Network.

Department of Health (2000) *Patient Group Directions* (England only) HSC 2000/026. London: Department of Health.

Department of Health (2002) *Health Check on the State of Public Health.* London: Annual Report of the Chief Medical Officer. Department of Health Publications.

Dodd ME et al. (2000) Audit of oxygen prescribing before and after the introduction of a prescription chart. *British Medical Journal* 321: 864–5.

Frazer RS, Crab R (2002) Dangers of hypoxia still greater than those of hyperoxia. (letter to the Editor), *British Medical Journal* 324: 1406.

Howell M (2001) An audit of oxygen prescribing in general medical wards. *Professional Nurse* 17(4): 221.

National Institute for Clinical Excellence (2004) *Chronic Obstructive Pulmonary Disease: Management of Chronic Obstructive Pulmonary Disease in Adults in Primary and Secondary Care.* Clinical Guideline 12. National Institute for Clinical Excellence.

O'Driscoll BR (2002) Oxygen therapy in acute medical care (letter to the Editor). *British Medical Journal* 324: 1406.

Small D et al. (1992) Uses and misuses of oxygen in hospitalised patients. *American Journal of Medicine* 92(6): 591–5.

Thompson AJ, Maxwell SRJ (2002) Oxygen therapy in acute medical care: the potential dangers of hyperoxia need to be recognised (editorial) *British Medical Journal* 324: 1406–7.

III Continuity of Care for the Critically Ill

7 Transferring patients from critical care to the ward

WAYNE ROBSON

INTRODUCTION

Since the mid 1990s health professionals have been encouraged to view critical illness in a more holistic way, with a beginning, a middle and an end. As a result there has been greater interest in the patient and relatives' experiences after they leave ICU or HDU, and in trying to ensure more seamless transfers to the wards. Continuity of care is increasingly something which patients and relatives see as important (Manley 1997). Both the Audit Commission Report *Critical to Success* (1999) and Department of Health document *Comprehensive Critical Care* (2000) recommended the introduction of critical care outreach teams. One of the main functions of these teams was to follow up patients who had been discharged from critical care to the wards. Prior to the introduction of critical care outreach teams patients and their relatives usually had no further contact with ICU or HDU after they had been transferred to the ward. It was hoped that outreach teams would provide some psychological support for patients and relatives in coping with the transition to the general ward, and in trying to make sense of their experience on critical care. Outreach teams also promised support for nurses on the wards in caring for acutely ill patients and those transferred from critical care. The introduction of critical care outreach teams has helped to raise awareness that for many patients and relatives the transfer to the ward is a daunting experience.

Patients who are moved from any familiar environment to a new and less familiar environment are known to find this process stressful, and this seems to apply equally to elderly patients moving from one nursing home to another, or to patients moving from intensive care or the high dependency unit to the ward. This type of stress has been referred to as 'relocation stress' or 'transfer anxiety'. However, it is not only the patients themselves who find this move stressful, but nursing staff and the patients' relatives may also be affected. This chapter will explore the above issues, and will

Critical Care Outreach. Edited by Lee Cutler and Wayne Robson.
Copyright 2006 by John Wiley & Sons Ltd.

review some of the key findings from the literature written on and around this topic. The aim of the chapter is to raise awareness about some of the complex issues surrounding the transfer of patients from critical care to the wards, and to explore how outreach nurses and those from the general wards and critical care can try to achieve well planned, safe and seamless transfers. The chapter will begin with a case study of a transfer that illustrates some of the individual, group and organisational barriers that can be encountered. The following points will then be discussed.

- What is relocation stress or transfer anxiety?
- What factors precipitate or worsen relocation stress?
- Why are seamless well-planned transfers from critical care important?
- A review of the literature relating to relocation stress and transfer anxiety after transfer from critical care.
- A review of the literature exploring the experiences of ward nurses caring for patients transferred from ICU.
- Tensions between ward nurses and critical care nurses. Is critical care nursing more stressful than general ward nursing?
- Recommendations for practice to ensure safe and seamless transfers from critical care.
- Barriers to implementing research recommendations designed to reduce relocation stress and promote seamless transfers.
- The role of the outreach team in ensuring safe seamless transfers.

CASE STUDY ILLUSTRATING THE POTENTIAL PITFALLS ENCOUNTERED IN TRANSFERS FROM CRITICAL CARE TO THE WARDS

Mr B is a 44-year-old man who has been on intensive care for the past four weeks. He has been extremely sick and has suffered from multi-organ failure as a result of severe sepsis secondary to pneumonia. He is now recovering and had his tracheostomy removed yesterday. He is still very weak and appears a little withdrawn and mildly confused. Today the intensive care unit is full, and there are two patients on the wards who need to be transferred to the unit. Mr B is the most appropriate patient for transfer. The plan was originally to send Mr B to the high dependency unit before transfer to the general ward, but HDU is full and it is felt that Mr B will be well enough to be managed on the ward. However before any planning and preparation can take place, one of the sick patients from the wards suffers a respiratory arrest and has to be brought to ICU immediately. Mr B is now transferred to the ward as quickly as possible (Box 7.1).

Box 7.1

As a result of emergency transfer:

- Mr B is not prepared for his move to the ward, and monitoring is abruptly removed
- ICU nursing staff feel frustrated that they are having to hurry Mr B out of ICU
- Mr B's relatives are suddenly informed that he is not going to HDU but is going directly to the ward in the next thirty minutes
- The bed manager tells one of the medical wards that they will be receiving Mr B from ICU

The ICU nurse arrives on the ward with Mr B. They are directed into one of the bays but nobody comes to greet them or to take a handover. After connecting Mr B up to the oxygen the ICU nurse goes to the nursing station to find the nurse who is going to take over Mr B's care. 'He has been really ill he had a swan ganz and has been on CVVH. Today his PO_2 was good and he has been cardiovascularly stable with just the occasional ectopic.' The ward nurse appears distracted, and unhappy about the timing of the transfer.

The ICU nurse finds it difficult to let go of the responsibility for Mr B as she has cared for him on a number of occasions over the past four weeks.

Box 7.2

- Communication between ICU and ward nurses is sometimes suboptimal, and ICU nurses may use language that can alienate ward staff
- Ward nurses find transfers from ICU stressful, and can as a result appear aloof
- Relatives feel scared that their loved one might deteriorate, and feel anxious that there are not enough staff on the ward
- Ward staff may not appreciate how weak and dependent ICU patients may be. Once free of all their lines and monitoring they may appear capable of doing more for themselves than they are actually able to do
- The handover from medical staff in critical care to the ward medical team is usually via a written discharge summary

That evening the healthcare assistant leaves an evening meal and a drink on Mr B's bedside table, unaware that he is very weak and has difficulty coordinating fine movements. As a result Mr B is unable to eat or drink very much.

Mr B's relatives visit and request to speak with a doctor. Today is Friday and there is only a junior doctor on call who is busy seeing other patients, and if she does become free she knows absolutely nothing about Mr B.

The critical care outreach service does not work weekends, and Mr B does not receive a follow-up visit until Monday, three days after his discharge from ICU. From the medical notes it appears that Mr B has not been reviewed over the weekend by a doctor.

The above case study reveals the varied and complex issues that can impact on the quality of transfers from critical care to the wards (Box 7.2).

WHAT IS RELOCATION STRESS OR TRANSFER ANXIETY?

The anxiety that patients can experience associated with transfer from ICU to the ward is commonly referred to in the literature as relocation stress or transfer anxiety (Box 7.3).

Relocation stress was accepted as a nursing diagnosis by the North American Nursing Diagnosis Association in 1992, and is defined by Carpenito (1995) as:

> a state in which an individual experiences physiologic and/or psychological disturbances as a result of transfer from one environment to another (p. 728).

Transfer anxiety, the other common name for relocation stress that tends to be used interchangeably, is defined by Roberts (1976) as:

> anxiety experienced by the individual when he/she moves from a familiar, somewhat secure environment to an environment that is unfamiliar (pp. 227–8).

Box 7.3 Signs and symptoms of relocation stress

- **Major characteristics:** loneliness, depression, anger, apprehension and anxiety
- **Minor characteristics:** changes in former eating and sleeping habits, dependency, insecurity, lack of trust and a need for excessive reassurance

Carpenito (2000)

WHAT FACTORS PRECIPITATE OR WORSEN RELOCATION STRESS

Relocation stress or transfer anxiety can be precipitated by the following events (Roberts 1976; Carpenito 1993, 1995):

* decreased physical health status;
* lack of preparation for transfer;
* significant degree of environmental change in the new environment;
* sudden reduction in patient monitoring;
* no explanation about the differences between critical care and the general wards;
* insufficient time to allow closure with the critical care staff;
* lack of predictability in the new environment;
* transfers that occur abruptly, during the night, or at shift handover times.

Patients on intensive care or high dependency are attached to lots of different pieces of equipment, ECG monitors, oxygen saturation probes, central venous pressure (CVP) and arterial lines, and their condition is monitored continuously. They also become used to having a nurse close by all the time. When the patient is transferred to the ward the monitoring may suddenly be discontinued and there will be a dramatic reduction in the nurse to patient ratio. Nurses on intensive care usually care for just one patient while nurses on the general wards commonly care for up to ten or more. If the patient is transferred to the ward in a hurry to create a bed for another admission then the monitoring may remain attached to the patient up until the moment the porter arrives to carry out the transfer. This abrupt removal of monitoring may make patients feel anxious and vulnerable. Why is it they can now manage without the monitors, when just five minutes earlier they seemed essential? A number of studies have recommended that monitoring should be gradually weaned from patients as their condition improves. This signals to the patient and his/her family that they are getting better and are in less need of such a high degree of care. Cutler and Garner (1995) point out that not all risk factors for relocation stress can be eliminated. One risk factor is decreased health status for example, but all patients leaving ICU will, by their very nature, have this. Another is a new and very different environment, something which the wards will always inevitably be after a stay in critical care.

WHY ARE SEAMLESS, WELL-PLANNED TRANSFERS FROM CRITICAL CARE IMPORTANT?

There are a number of reasons why well-planned seamless transfers from critical care are important. Probably the most significant of these is that poorly planned transfers put patients at risk, and can potentially increase a patient's mortality and morbidity. Failure to pass on information about tests or medications a patient may have had or may need, for example, could have serious consequences. Ball (2005) argues that the risks involved in transfer from intensive care are multi-faceted and will be affected by the patient's age, any residual organ dysfunction they may have, their length of stay on ICU, and poor communication between critical care and the wards. Separate episodes of care delivered to the patient in different areas of the hospital need to join together smoothly so that the patient's journey to recovery is uninterrupted. This joining together of various episodes of care is about continuity. Manley (1997) argues that continuity of care is

> an indicator of quality related to improved outcomes, a more personalized service for users, cost effective use of healthcare resources, and job satisfaction for healthcare professionals. (p. 265)

Patients who are transferred from ICU to the ward are still in the process of recovering from their critical illness, and some of these patients will not survive to be discharged from hospital. Others may suffer a deterioration in their condition, and a small number of these may require readmission to either ICU or HDU. Patients who are over 70 years of age and those who have had a stay on ICU longer than 6.5 days are thought to be most at risk of readmission (Metnitz et al. 2003).

Patients who are readmitted to ICU are known to have a high mortality. It is essential then that there is effective communication and planning to reduce any potential risks to the patients' continued recovery.

Aside from the obvious benefits of well-planned transfers for the patients' well-being, it can also have dramatic effects on the patients' and relatives' experience.

The patients' and relatives' experience of care is becoming increasingly more important. As health professionals we are encouraged to listen to the patients' and relatives' experiences, through satisfaction questionnaires and discovery interviews. One of the things patients value highly as part of a good experience is effective communication. This includes both direct communication to them personally and communication about them between health professionals, and healthcare organisations. Poor communication is frequently one of the reasons that patients choose to complain about their experience in hospital. Good communication is essential to help ensure the patient and relatives have a positive experience of being transferred from ICU to the ward.

PATIENTS' EXPERIENCES FOLLOWING TRANSFER FROM INTENSIVE CARE

A number of studies have explored the patients' experience of transferring to the ward. The findings of three recent UK studies will be briefly discussed.

In 1997 a study by Hall-Smith et al. interviewed 26 patents who had attended an intensive-care follow-up outpatient clinic. Patients reported that they often felt unobserved and vulnerable on the ward.

Odell (2000) interviewed six patients who had been transferred from intensive care to the ward. This study revealed that the patients' reaction to transfer can be 'complex and often interwoven with different conflicting emotions' (p. 328).

Patients in this study had a mixture of feelings about their transfer, some positive and some negative. Indifferent and ambivalent feelings were expressed, but upon deeper discussion patients revealed conflicting emotions. Some of the patients could not remember much about their transfer. Odell (2000) suggests that the feelings of indifference and the poor memory of events may be the result of as yet unexplored feelings, or denial of events as a coping mechanism.

Patients revealed that they found the transfer tiring, and that they forgot some of the information they were told about the transfer. Odell (2000) states that patients being transferred from ICU therefore need to have information about their transfer reinforced and updated.

McKinney and Deeny (2002), in what appear to be one of the most recent studies exploring patients' experiences of being transferred from ICU, interviewed six patients. The patients were interviewed on ICU pre-transfer and then again on the ward post-transfer. Like Odell (2000) this study revealed mixed feelings among patients regarding transfer; however, four of the six patients viewed the transfer in a negative light. Most of the patients made reference to physical problems such as weakness or limited mobility, and some felt frustrated by their slow progress: 'I feel I'm not coming on . . . Not getting better as quick as I should' (p. 327).

Many of the patients mentioned the difficulty they experienced adjusting to the lower staff ratios on the ward, and the loss of the close relationship they enjoyed with staff while on ICU.

McKinney and Deeny (2002) make a number of recommendations. Many of these have been made in earlier studies. They suggest discussing transfer with patients and informing them about what to expect. Gradually reducing monitoring and level of attention before transfer takes place. Providing education for ward nurses to ensure they are aware of the physical and psychological needs of patients post-transfer. They also stress that not all patients transferring from ICU will experience relocation stress, and that therefore a blanket diagnosis of relocation stress is not appropriate to apply to all (Box 7.4).

McKinney and Deeny (2002) argue that critical care outreach may be able to reduce the stress of transfer. It appears that at the time of writing no studies have evaluated the effects of outreach in reducing the stress patients can experience after transfer from ICU to the ward.

Box 7.4 Key messages

• Not all patients experience relocation stress. An individualised approach should be used that identifies and targets those at greatest risk

• Patients may not remember information they are given on ICU about the transfer

• Information regarding transfer must therefore be repeated and reinforced

---

RELATIVES' EXPERIENCES FOLLOWING TRANSFER OF THEIR LOVED ONE FROM ICU

Relocation stress can also be experienced by the relatives of patients who are transferred from ICU to a general ward. Streater et al. (2001) explored the relocation experiences of relatives leaving a neurosciences ICU. Relatives found the lower staff ratios on the wards difficult to adjust to:

> I hope that they [the ward staff] will be able to keep an eye on him. (p. 166)

Some of the relatives felt that the ward staff could sometimes appear aloof or impersonal. Streater et al. (2001) suggested that this may be a coping mechanism used by staff to survive stressful events, such as the transfer of a patient from ICU to a busy ward.

Relatives identified inadequate information at the time of transfer as a major cause of anxiety. Streater et al. (2001) recommended that patients and relatives should receive a welcome and introduction from the ward staff when they arrive, and that ward staff should try to meet the patient and their relatives before the actual transfer takes place.

An information booklet about the transfer to be given to relatives while on ICU was also recommended.

RECOMMENDATIONS FOR PRACTICE TO ENSURE SAFE, SEAMLESS TRANSFERS FROM CRITICAL CARE

Leith (1998) summarised the 20 most commonly suggested nursing interventions for transfer anxiety or relocation stress that appear in the nursing literature. The most frequently suggested interventions were some of the following (see also Figure 7.1).

- Recognising the potential for relocation stress.
- Comparing and contrasting the general ward and intensive care.
- Following a structured teaching plan for discharge to the ward.
- Interpreting the transfer as a positive sign.
- Introducing the patient to the nurse on the ward who will be receiving them.
- Encouraging patients to talk about the transfer and ask questions.
- Written information explaining what to expect after transfer to the ward. Research suggests that patients may be given some verbal explanations about their transfer while still on ICU but that they may not remember receiving such information (Odell 2000; Paul et al. 2004). Information booklets are therefore recommended to reinforce verbal explanations (Streater et al. 2001; Paul et al. 2004). Gradually reducing the level of observation and care as the patient's condition improves. One example of this strategy might be to remove monitoring leads gradually in readiness for transfer (Coyle 2001; McKinney and Deeny 2002).
- Educational sessions for nurses on the wards to promote a greater aware-ness of the physiological and psychological problems commonly encoun-tered in post-critical care patients (McKinney and Deeny 2002; Robson 2003).
- Paying attention to any coping constraints that the patient may have. These are things like pain and fatigue that if not addressed may weaken the patient's ability to cope with stress (Bokinskie 1992). Cutler and Garner (1995) state that because each patient will react individually to their trans-fer from ICU, their preparation therefore needs to be individualised.
- Improved discharge planning on ICU.
- Collaboration and liaison between critical care nurses and ward nurses (Coyle 2001).

TENSIONS BETWEEN WARD NURSES AND CRITICAL CARE NURSES

As early as 1989 conflict between ICU and non-ICU nurses was referred to in the American nursing literature. In this particular study Schultz and Daly (1989) state that the two groups of staff 'sometimes create a milieu for con-flict'. Common reasons for such conflict include the timing of transfers from ICU to the ward, equipment needs, communication, and questions about whether the patient is ready for transfer to the ward (Figure 7.2).

Language can also be a source of problems. Hall-Smith et al. (1997) suggest that the use of words such as 'stable' by ICU staff are subjective and open to misinterpretation, and saying a patient has 'done very well' can 'lead to a false sense of security for ward staff' (p. 247).

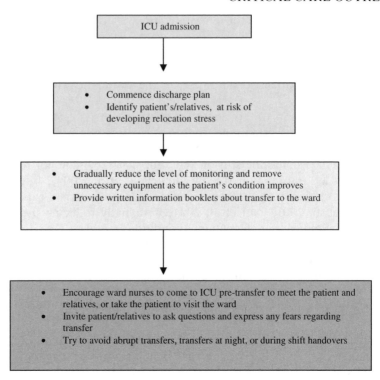

Figure 7.1 A structured approach to preparing patients and relatives for transfer to the ward.

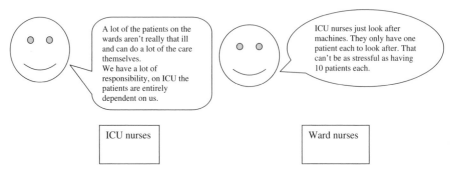

Figure 7.2 Tensions between ward nurses and critical care nurses.

When handing over a patient to the ward staff critical care nurses should avoid too much detail about aspects of care from ICU or HDU such as mechanical ventilation and inotropes and should stress that although the patient is stable, and doing well they are still at high risk of deterioration, and require close observation. Hall-Smith et al. (1997) redesigned discharge documentation to make it more relevant and meaningful to ward staff, detailing the patient's physical ability and how much care they required.

Schultz and Daly (1989) argue that the conflict between ICU and non-ICU nurses is the result of stereotypes each group of nurses hold about the other and the perceptions each group may hold that their area of nursing is harder work or more stressful.

A number of studies have explored whether it is more stressful to work on an intensive care unit or on a non-intensive care unit. Boumans and Landeweerd (1994) state that although there may be a widely held assumption that nursing in ICU is more stressful than on the general ward areas this has not been confirmed by research findings.

One way of breaking down such stereotypes is to encourage nurses from critical care and the general wards to spend some time working in each other's areas so that both then gain some appreciation of each other's pressures.

THE EXPERIENCES OF WARD NURSES CARING FOR PATIENTS TRANSFERRED FROM ICU

In 1995 a study by Cutler and Garner surveyed nurses from six wards in a district general hospital to try to identify any problems they encountered with patient transfers from ICU. The ward nurses raised concerns about the stress that patients manifested upon transfer and the lack of awareness patients had about their workload on the wards. Many of them thought the idea of ward nurses visiting the patient in ICU prior to their transfer was a good one. Many of the problems identified by the ward nurses could, suggest Cutler and Garner (1995), be resolved by improved communication between the staff in ICU and the receiving ward.

In the last five years two studies from the UK have specifically explored in greater depth the experiences of ward nurses in caring for patients transferred from intensive care (Whittaker and Ball 2000; Haines et al. 2001). The main findings of these two studies will now be discussed.

Both studies found that ward nurses find accepting transfers from ICU stressful. In Haines et al. (2001) all participants referred to the stress, anxiety or fear that was experienced when a patient was accepted from ICU. One participant commented, 'Receiving these people [ICU patients] back, is often quite daunting' (p. 19).

In Whitaker and Ball's (2000) study junior nurses expressed a sense of dread, or described feeling depressed when finding out that they were to receive a patient from ICU.

Ward nurses in Haines et al. (2001) felt that they had little control over the transfer process, and talked of the difficulties in trying to care for a transfer from ICU while also trying to care for the rest of their allocated patients. One respondent commented, 'They're bedbound, they've got . . . catheters, CVPs and whatever, and they come back needing you and by the time you've sorted them out it's more or less time to repeat the process' (p. 19).

Patients from ICU were seen as being very demanding, expecting the nurses to do everything for them, and were referred to as being 'institution-alised' and 'buzzer happy' (p. 20). It was not revealed in the study whether ward nurses were aware that this demanding behaviour may have been a manifestation of relocation stress. This finding might also suggest that ward nurses are not fully aware of the profound degree of muscle loss some ICU patients undergo (Griffiths and Jones 1999), leaving them extremely weak and unable to carry out even simple tasks unaided.

In both studies ward nurses talked about the anxieties of relatives upon transfer to the ward. They were concerned about the level of care their relative would receive in a busy general ward environment. In Haines et al. (2001) ward nurses also describe the difficulties in providing psychological support to post ICU patients who were often frightened and vulnerable.

Both studies suggested that ward nurses sometimes felt that communication between ICU and the wards was sub-optimal. Some of the participants in Whitaker and Ball (2000) displayed some negative feelings about the verbal handover from ICU nurses, pointing out that it was often too detailed: 'they were talking about metabolic acidosis and blood gas results that happened three days ago . . . it could be put on more friendly terms' (p. 139).

The ward nurses in both studies felt that ICU nurses could do more to prepare patients for transfer to the ward. In particular making sure that the patient and their relatives were aware of the differences in staffing levels between the two areas. The findings of Whittaker and Ball (2000) and Haines et al. (2001) suggest that despite a number of published studies over the past twenty years recommending a variety of interventions to reduce relocation stress, in practice such recommendations may not always be acted upon. The possible reasons why the adoption of these recommendations appears slow will be explored in the next section of this chapter.

A summary of the main recommendations from Whittaker and Ball (2000) and Haines et al. (2001) is given in Table 7.1.

BARRIERS TO IMPLEMENTING RESEARCH RECOMMENDATIONS TO REDUCE RELOCATION STRESS AND PROMOTE SEAMLESS TRANSFERS

One of the barriers appears to be that nurses on ICU do not always see discharge planning as being very important, or as being within the remit of crit-

Table 7.1 Summary of recommendations

Whittaker and Ball (2000)	Haines et al. (2001)
ICU nurses to have more understanding of the ward nurses' workload	Proactive discharge planning in ICU
Give ward nurses prior warning of any equipment needed	More control for ward nurses regarding information about transfers
Education for both ward nurses and ICU nurses about discharge	Increasing knowledge of relocation stress
Relatives to visit the ward prior to discharge	Follow-up support from ICU
Ward staff to be invited to meet the patient in ICU prior to discharge	Pre-transfer visit to ICU from ward nurse

ical care. Schlemmer (1989) found that many critical care nurses thought discharge planning in ICU was not practical, and they did not regard it as a priority. Whitaker and Ball (2000) point out that since the above study by Schlemmer (1989) few studies on discharge planning in ICU have been carried out, possibly indicating that it is a subject that is not regarded as a high priority. Leith (1998) suggests that one way of improving discharge planning in ICU would be to integrate it into a care pathway or protocol.

Relocation stress is not a new concept, and since the early 1980s there have been articles published highlighting this as a problem initially for patients leaving the coronary care unit (Poe 1982; Schactman 1987). However, many nurses on ICU and the general wards may be unaware of the findings of these early studies carried out in CCU, and the more recent publications exploring ICU patients' experiences of transfer (Odell 2000), and those of ward nurses receiving such transfers (Whittaker and Ball 2000). If nurses are not aware of relocation stress they cannot begin to prevent it.

Lack of beds on ICU relative to demand often means transfers from critical care occur in a hurried fashion to make a bed available for another patient (Robson 2004). This means that there is less opportunity to prepare the patients and relatives. Monitoring cannot be removed gradually and the differences between the general wards and ICU cannot be discussed. Although the number of ICU beds has increased significantly since 2000, it appears that the number of beds is still often not sufficient to meet demand. When compared with other European countries and the United States, hospitals in the United Kingdom have very low numbers of ICU beds. The figure generally quoted is that 1% of total hospital beds are ICU beds. In a recent unpublished study (Robson 2004) critical care nurses felt that they were still sometimes having to rush patients out of critical care to the wards to make beds available for other sick patients awaiting admission.

In the past fifteen years patients on the wards have become older and more acutely ill (Anderson 1999). One of the reasons for this is the growth of day-case surgery, or day-case medical procedures. Previously the patient population on the wards would have included some patients having investigations or minor surgery. This group of patients now have these procedures performed as day cases, which means that the remaining patients on the wards are more likely to be acutely ill or undergoing major surgery. The increased acuity on the general wards and lack of staff limit the opportunity for ward nurses to come to ICU pre-transfer to meet the patient and their relatives.

Whittaker and Ball (2001) highlight that recommendations from previous studies on relocation stress concentrate on ways in which it might be reduced without paying attention to the workload of ward nurses.

Box 7.5 Barriers to implementing research recommendations

- Insufficient critical care beds to meet demand
- Discharge planning often occurs too late
- Ward nurses are often unable to meet ICU patients pre-transfer because the high workload and patient acuity on the general wards makes it hard for them to be released
- Junior staff on ICU may be unaware of research on relocation stress and what they can do to prevent it

---

THE ROLE OF THE OUTREACH TEAM IN ENSURING SAFE AND SEAMLESS TRANSFERS

As has already been discussed in this chapter, there are two groups of nurses involved in the transfer process from critical care to the wards, and these groups can often appear to be polarised. Critical care outreach nurses are in a unique position to act as a bridge to unify and galvanise the two camps in the pursuit of evidence-based, safe and seamless transfers. One of the key roles of outreach is education, and this should include teaching critical care nurses and ward nurses about relocation stress and the findings and recommendations of studies such as Cutler and Garner (1995), Whittaker and Ball (2000) and Haines et al. (2001).

A recent study by Richardson et al. (2004) explored ward nurses' evaluation of critical care outreach. Ward nurses were very positive in their evaluation and commented that they found 'the feedback and joint communication very helpful' (p. 33) when outreach nurses came to the ward to visit patients after transfer. When asked how outreach could be improved, a common theme was the feeling that the service should be available 24 hours a day.

One argument for having a 24-hour outreach service is that some patients are discharged from ICU outside of normal office hours, a percentage of these occurring at night. A study by Goldfrad and Rowan (2000) showed that patients discharged at night fare significantly worse than patients who are discharged during the day. The presence of outreach at night may facilitate communication between ICU and the wards and would mean that the ward nurses have access to support and advice outside of office hours when there are also fewer medical staff around.

To justify the cost of extending outreach services to 24 hours, there would have to be very strong evidence that it makes a difference. This evidence would need to be in terms of improving patient survival, reduction of cardiac arrests and readmissions to ICU or HDU. Evidence is now beginning to emerge that outreach may improve survival to hospital discharge and reduce readmissions to critical care (Ball et al. 2003; Priestly et al. 2004).

As well as visiting patients on the wards after transfer, outreach teams also need to be involved in ICU and HDU with discharge planning. One example of this is discharge planning for tracheostomy patients.

At Chesterfield Royal Hospital (UK) critical care outreach nurses arrange multi-disciplinary meetings between ward nurses, outreach, physiotherapy, speech and language therapy to formulate a discharge plan for patients being transferred to the ward with a tracheostomy. The outreach team provide training for ward nurses on all aspects of tracheostomy care and ensure that the necessary equipment is in place prior to the transfer.

Outreach nurses could also be involved in efforts to reduce the risks of patients developing relocation stress by arranging for ward nurses to visit ICU to meet the patient and family, or by taking the patient in a chair with their family to meet the nurses on the ward where they are being transferred to.

SUMMARY

Critical care outreach teams can play an important role in helping to ensure safe, seamless and well-planned transfers from critical care to the wards. They can achieve this in the following ways:

- helping to break down stereotypes that ward nurses and critical care nurses sometimes hold about each other;
- inviting and facilitating ward nurses to visit patients in ICU before the patients transfer;
- disseminating research findings on relocation stress, physical and psychological problems post-ICU, discharge planning and transfers, between staff in the two areas.

Although critical care outreach teams can have some influence over the quality of transfers, in order for the recommendations of previous studies to be successfully put into practice more resources also appear to be needed.

This should include an increased number of critical care beds and a review of the staffing levels on the wards with a view to increasing them to reflect the increase in the number of acutely ill patients on the general wards that has occurred since the early 1990s.

SUGGESTED READING/KEY TEXTS

Ball C (2005) Ensuring a successful discharge from intensive care. *Intensive and Critical Care Nursing* 21: 1–4.

Haines S, Crocker C, Leducq M (2001) Providing continuity of care for patients transferred from ICU. *Professional Nurse* 17(1): 17–21.

Leith BA (1998) Transfer anxiety in critical care patients and their family members. *Critical Care Nurse* 18: 4, 24–32.

McKinney AA, Melby V (2002) Relocation stress in critical care: a review of the literature. *Journal of Clinical Nursing* 11: 149–57.

Whittaker J, Ball C (2000) Discharge from intensive care: a view from the ward. *Intensive and Critical Care Nursing* 16: 135–43.

REFERENCES

Anderson ID (ed.) (1999) *Care of the Critically Ill Surgical Patient*. London: Arnold.

Audit Commission (1999) *Critical to Success: The Place of Efficient and Effective Critical Care Services within the Acute Hospital*. London: Audit Commission.

Ball C (2005) Ensuring a successful discharge from intensive care. *Intensive and Critical Care Nursing* 21: 1–4.

Ball C, Kirkby M, Williams S (2003) Effects of the critical care outreach team on patient survival to discharge from hospital and readmissions to critical care: a non-randomised population study. *British Medical Journal* 327: 1014–17.

Bokinskie JC (1992) Family conferences: a method to diminish transfer anxiety. *Journal of Neurosciences Nursing* 24: 129–33.

Boumans NPG, Landeweerd JA (1994) Working in an intensive or non intensive care unit: Does it make any difference? *Heart & Lung* 23: 1, 71–9.

Carpenito LJ (1993) *Nursing Diagnosis: Application to Clinical Practice* 5th edn. Philadelphia: Lippincott.

Carpenito LJ (1995) *Nursing Diagnosis: Application to Clinical Practice* 6th edn. Philadelphia: Lippincott.

Carpenito LJ (2000) *Nursing Diagnosis: Application to Clinical Practice* 8th edn. Philadelphia: Lippincott.

Coyle MA (2001) Transfer anxiety: preparing to leave intensive care. *Intensive and Critical Care Nursing* 17: 138–43.

Cutler L, Garner M (1995) Reducing relocation stress after discharge from the intensive therapy unit. *Intensive and Critical Care Nursing* 11: 333–5.

Department of Health (2000) *Comprehensive Critical Care: A Review of Adult Critical Care Services*. London: Department of Health.

Goldfrad C, Rowan K (2000) Consequences of discharges from intensive care at night. *The Lancet* 355: 1138–42.

Griffiths RD, Jones C (1999) Recovery from intensive care. *British Medical Journal* 319: 427–9.

Haines S, Crocker C, Leducq M (2001) Providing continuity of care for patients transferred from ICU. *Professional Nurse* 17(1): 17–21.

Hall-Smith J, Ball C, Coakley J (1997) Follow up services and the development of a clinical nurse specialist in intensive care. *Intensive and Critical Care Nursing* 13: 243–8.

Leith BA (1998) Transfer anxiety in critical care patients and their family members. *Critical Care Nurse* 18(4): 24–32.

McKinney AA, Deeny P (2002) Leaving the intensive care unit: a phenomenological study of the patient's experience. *Intensive and Critical Care Nursing* 18: 320–31.

McKinney AA, Melby V (2002) Relocation stress in critical care: a review of the literature. *Journal of Clinical Nursing* 11: 149–57.

Manley K (1997) Continuity of care: what is the nurse's role in critical care. *Nursing in Critical Care* 2(6): 265–6.

Metnitz PG, Fieux F, Jordan B et al. (2003) Critically ill patients readmitted to intensive care units – lessons to learn. *Intensive Care Medicine* 29: 241–8.

Odell M (2000) The patients' thoughts and feelings about their transfer from intensive care to the general ward. *Journal of Advanced Nursing* 31(2): 322–9.

Paul F, Hendry C, Cabrelli L (2004) Meeting patient and relatives' information needs upon transfer from an intensive care unit: the development and evaluation of an information booklet. *Journal of Clinical Nursing* 13: 396–405.

Poe CM (1982) Minimizing stress of transfer responses. *Dimensions of Critical Care Nursing* 1: 364–74.

Priestly G, Watson W, Rashidan A et al. (2004) Introducing critical care outreach: a ward randomised trial of phased introduction in a general hospital. *Intensive Care Medicine* 30: 1398–1404.

Richardson A, Burnard V, Colley H et al. (2004) Ward nurses' evaluation of critical care outreach. *Nursing in Critical Care* 9(1): 28–33.

Roberts SL (1976) Transfer anxiety. In: *Behavioural Concepts and the Critically Ill Patient*, pp. 224–52. Englewood Cliffs, NJ: Prentice Hall.

Robson WP (2003) The physiological after effects of critical care. *Nursing in Critical Care* 8(4): 165–71.

Robson WP (2004) The experiences of critical care nurses and ward nurses on caring for patients transferring from intensive care, and high dependency units to the general wards. Unpublished MSc thesis. Sheffield Hallam University.

Schactman M (1987) Transfer stress in patients after MI. *Focus Critical Care* 14(2): 34–7.

Schlemmer B (1989) The status of discharge planning in intensive care units. *Nursing Management* 20: 7, 88A–88P.

Schultz MA, Daly B (1989) Differences and similarities in nurses' perceptions of intensive care nursing and non-intensive care nursing. *Focus on Critical Care* 16(6): 465–71.

Streater C, Golledge J, Sutherland H et al. (2001) The relocation experiences of relatives leaving a neurosciences critical care unit: a phenomenological study. *Nursing in Critical Care* 6(4): 163–70.

Whittaker J, Ball C (2000) Discharge from intensive care: a view from the ward. *Intensive and Critical Care Nursing* 16: 135–43.

8 Critical care outreach follow-up

KATE BRAY

INTRODUCTION

An episode of critical illness and admission to a critical care unit does not start and end exclusively in the critical care environment. The critically ill patient requires physical, psychological and emotional care to be provided as part of a care pathway into the community and home. Previous chapters have highlighted the role of the outreach nurse in supporting acutely ill patients before admission to critical care, the continuation of the patient's journey can also be enhanced by critical care outreach after discharge from critical care to the ward. The Audit Commission Report, *Critical to Success* (Audit Commission 1999), was the most comprehensive examination of critical care services in England and Wales since the evolution of this speciality. It included an emphasis on quality of life after an admission to intensive care, and made several recommendations:

- To focus research on both survival and long-term effects of survivors.
- Liaise with primary care and admitting consultants to provide rehabilitation services that meet the particular needs of ex-critical care patients, especially those who have been sedated for ventilation. If necessary, a specialist follow-up clinic service and a rehabilitation programme should be considered.
- Use a standard assessment procedure before discharge to identify those patients who are most likely to be in need of specialist rehabilitation due to their stay in critical care.

The focus of this chapter is to discuss the role critical care outreach has in meeting the follow-up needs of intensive care patients. Current knowledge of the outcomes of intensive care survivors will be discussed, and the challenges to the outreach nurse in addressing this part of the outreach service.

BACKGROUND

The concept of quality of life and outcomes after an admission to intensive care is not new. While the early years of intensive care had focused on patient survival, by the 1980s and 1990s the concept of examining the outcomes along the continuum from critical illness through to physical and psychological rehabilitation grew. Prior to the Audit Commission Report (Audit Commission 1999) previous reports had highlighted the need for enquiry into long-term survival and outcomes of intensive care patients (Association of Anaesthetists 1988; Metcalf and McPherson 1995). The interest in examining outcomes from intensive care is stimulated by continuing technological and medical advances, chronic illness, and an increasingly elderly population, alongside scarce resources and the cost effectiveness of treatments. Examination of such issues is now an accepted part of intensive care evaluation, nationally and internationally, and a systematic review of such evidence has been compiled (Hayes and Black 2000; Angus and Carlet 2003). Much has already been investigated and written about in regard to the follow-up of patients from intensive care, and is well illustrated (Griffiths and Jones 2002). Patients' knowledge, perceptions and expectations of health care have also emerged over the last decade. Department of Health policy now states that 'the patient and service user must come first' (DoH 2004b). Griffiths and Jones (2002) suggest that the very essence of intensive care follow-up is to develop our knowledge about intensive care practice, and so ensure the well-being of intensive care patients.

Following the Audit Commission Report (1999), the expert critical care group, established by the Department of Health to propose a framework for adult critical care services in the future (DoH 2000), recommended that NHS Trusts should review the provision of follow-up services and ensure that there is provision for such.

CRITICAL CARE OUTREACH AND FOLLOW-UP CARE

In the United Kingdom about 60% of hospital admissions are emergencies (Bion and Heffner 2004). Some of the difficulties in caring for such acutely ill patients in hospitals today are attributed to an ever-increasing throughput of patients, unpredictable workloads, and the uncertainty about the course of illness in individual patients. Critical care outreach has been described as 'one of the success stories of the modernisation of critical care' (DoH 2003), as the emphasis of this service is to share critical care skills with ward staff, and support the acutely ill patient before and after an admission to a critical care unit. There is now plentiful evidence to demonstrate that sub-optimal general ward care is associated with increased mortality (McGloin et al. 1997; McQuillan et al. 1998).

It may appear that the emphasis of critical care outreach is to care for those patients whose condition is at risk of deteriorating in the ward areas, to avoid an admission to critical care. However part of the whole outreach service is also described as:

> To enable discharges by supporting the continuing recovery of discharged patients on the wards, and post discharge from hospital, and their relatives and friends. (DoH 2000)

This is revisited in the National Outreach Report (DoH 2003) as one of the key features of outreach work is seen as post-critical care discharge follow-up in hospital.

For the clinicians working in intensive care, in an ideal world patients would remain in a unit until their condition was optimum; however, due to lack of beds some are discharged before this optimal point, often in an emergency when a bed is needed for another sick patient. Evidence has shown that 9–16% of discharges from critical care will be re-admitted due to a recurrence of their initial disease (Goldhill and Sumner 1998). Indeed the outcomes of patients discharged from intensive care at night have been found to be worse than those discharged to general wards during the day (Goldfrad and Rowan 2000). High dependency can act as step-down units, and would facilitate continued rehabilitation, particularly for patients who have been in intensive care for some time. However, with the ever-increasing demand and pressure for critical care beds, patients may be discharged to a general ward sooner than anticipated. It is evident that critical care outreach needs to monitor the progress of all critical care discharges in case of a deterioration of their condition in general ward areas. Once the acute phase diminishes, with regard to ongoing rehabilitation it is suggested that critical care outreach is best placed to continue to monitor the condition of such patients, and offer support in their ongoing care (Griffiths and Jones 2002).

In the initial visits to patients after leaving critical care, the emphasis will be on their acute condition. This may include assessing physiological and fluid balance status, ongoing drug therapy, and any other support patient and ward staff may require with venous lines and tracheostomy. However, at the same time the patient will need support, advice, reassurance and explanations of care received while in critical care, and ongoing therapy.

Enquiry and research into the outcomes of intensive care outcomes began in the late 1970s, with many studies looking at long-term mortality rates up to five years (Keenan et al. 2004). This information however only informs of survival rates, and the authors suggest that information on quality of life for these survivors is as necessary to inform intensive care practice. Research and evaluation of recovering critically ill patients from the 1980s onwards have demonstrated that after an episode of critical illness patients can be left with the following problems.

NEUROMUSCULAR WEAKNESS AND FUNCTIONAL PROBLEMS

An episode of critical illness can cause a loss of to up to 2% of muscle mass per day. This leads to severe muscle wasting, weakness, fatigue and difficulty in swallowing and coughing (Ridley 2002). Indeed muscle weakness is described as the 'most obvious and debilitating feature of recovery from critical illness' (Griffiths and Jones 2002, p. 8). This is often described as critical illness polyneuropathy and may be accompanied by numbness and paraesthesia, patients describe a physical weakness that prevents them from carrying out many normal care activities. It is suggested that poor functional status, and a subsequent physical recovery from critical illness can take many months if not years (Gardner and Sibthorpe 2002; Angus and Carlet 2003).

NUTRITIONAL PROBLEMS

As previously described, critically ill patients can lose large amounts of muscle mass during critical illness (Griffiths and Jones 2002). Combined with fatigue, loss of appetite, changes in taste and weakness, it is a challenge for such patients to maintain an adequate diet to recover weight lost. Patients may have difficulties in swallowing due to weakness and tracheostomy scarring. The high emphasis on adequate nutrition and monitoring intake that occurs in the critical care unit must continue in the ward area, with continued input from the dietetic teams.

PSYCHOLOGICAL PROBLEMS

Many studies have shown that that ICU survivors are more likely to suffer post-traumatic stress disorder, anxiety and depression, which relates to a poor quality of life physically and mentally (Jones et al. 1998, 2001; Skirrow et al. 2001; Angus and Carlet 2003). Such studies have informed us that the critical care patients may suffer from memory loss, nightmares, hallucinations, sleep disturbance, unpleasant memories of critical care, anxiety and depression. Some patients have little memory or recall of an admission to critical care, and may yet have vivid dreams and nightmares that are upsetting and disturb-ing to the individual.

Patients may report many other symptoms related to their critical illness and original diagnosis. Other physical problems reported from follow-up clinics are painful joints, dry skin and changes to skin and nails, intolerance to cold/heat, bowel dysfunction, hair loss, altered taste and sexual dysfunction (Griffiths and Jones 2002; Sheffield Teaching Hospitals 2003).

CAREGIVER BURDEN

The long-term effect of critical illness on close family and caregivers of patients is now being understood as more follow-up of critical care patients occurs (Johnson et al. 2001; Angus and Carlet 2003). Such families have witnessed and had to cope with the crisis of their loved one going through a critical illness. It has been found that relatives of these patients can also suffer from symptoms of anxiety, depression and post-traumatic stress disorder (Skirrow et al. 2001).

The previous description of physical and psychological effects of critical illness, and potential effects on patients' families, require the critical care outreach nurse to be competent and confident in supporting the rehabilitation of such patients in the ward areas. Critical care outreach nurses need to be experienced in caring for critically ill patients, and understanding of the critical care environments, in order to manage ongoing physical and psychological problems of the patients. Patients and their families will have questions and queries about past and current care. To offer guidance and support for this the critical care outreach nurse needs to have the ability to counsel and advise patients. They also need to be able to identify when patients need more specialist psychological help, and be able to refer on accordingly. The scope, abilities and expectations of critical care outreach nurses need to be part of ongoing individual development, to ensure these specialist posts can follow up and support patients in the general wards.

Ideally an individual patient rehabilitation programme needs to start in the critical care unit and must be monitored by critical care outreach for continuity of care. Better outcomes were demonstrated in patients who received a rehabilitation package, against those who did not, in a randomised control trial (Jones et al. 2003). In following up critical care patients, to ensure comprehensive and continued care, critical care outreach nurses must have the autonomy to refer and liaise with other members of the multi-disciplinary team, such as physiotherapists, dieticians and other specialist professionals, to optimise the recovery of these patients. Educational programmes for ward staff, while aimed at managing the acutely ill patient, need to include the physical and psychological problems patients face after critical care. General ward staff with no experience of working in critical care will be generally unaware of the effects of critical illness and how it can impact upon the rehabilitation and recovery of these patients. At this point outreach plays a crucial role in the care pathway from critical care to the ward, and into the community.

FORMAL FOLLOW-UP CLINICS

The concept of a follow-up clinic after intensive care is not new. At Whiston Hospital in Liverpool such a clinic has been in operation since 1990. Many hospitals have established formal critical care follow-up clinics, and their benefits have been widely demonstrated (Audit Commission 1999; Griffiths and Jones 2002; Crocker 2003). The difficulties establishing such a clinic and measuring valid outcomes are well described by Crocker (2003). The process to establish this clinic took nine months of background preparation; this is reflected in the author's experience locally (Sheffield Teaching Hospitals 2003). Establishing ongoing funding from stretched budgets can be a difficult issue. It is suggested that the cost of a doctor-led multi-disciplinary clinic with administrative support is approximately £30,000 (Griffiths and Jones 2002), while a nurse-led service may be more economical. Crocker (2003) found that patients suffered from reduced mobility, physical weakness and psychological problems, as confirmed in other follow-up. This follow-up clinic also found that other feedback from patients and their families on the service they received in hospital was valuable, enforcing the need to start the process of rehabilitation in the critical care units. Gaps in service regarding discharge home and into the community were found. Similar findings were also demonstrated from a pilot of a follow-up clinic, where gaps in care in the patients' pathway were identified, and a plan of action developed to improve this (unpublished data: Pilot of an Intensive Care Follow up Clinic, Sheffield Teaching Hospitals 2003).

EXPERIENCES FROM A PILOT STUDY FOLLOW-UP CLINIC

During the six-month pilot in a large tertiary referral teaching hospital, 70 patients were seen three months after discharge from intensive care, from two hospital sites, and two intensive care units. Within this hospital trust both hospitals have separate intensive care units. Prior to starting the clinic, nursing staff contacted other intensive care units known to have follow-up clinics, and found the criteria for offering patients an appointment varied according to the length of time patients had been ventilated from 2 to 4 days. As the majority of admissions to the dedicated intensive care units are ventilated, all 177 patients who had been admitted to these units over a six-month period were invited to attend.

NON-ATTENDANCE AND ALTERNATIVE FOLLOW-UP TO CLINICS

One of the main problems faced by clinic nurses initially was the number of patients who did not attend or who rang to cancel the appointment. Forty-two patients who did not attend or cancelled had an admission in intensive care of less than 48 hours. Other units who had established follow-up clinics were contacted for advice, and confirmed that general non-attendance was a problem they also faced. To address the problem of non-attendance the clinic nurses telephoned patients to ask if they would like an appointment. At this point, three months after discharge from intensive care, some patients felt physically unable to attend, but did want to discuss problems and ask questions via the telephone. This method of follow-up could be considered as a preferred method for some patients, particularly if funding of a formal clinic is difficult. For other patients appointments times and dates were agreed by phone, ensuring patients were offered choice of attendance convenient to them. This method is advocated to improve DNA rates and service delivery by the NHS Modernisation Agency (DoH 2004a).

OUTCOME MEASURES

To examine physical and psychological outcomes the following well-validated assessment tools were used in the clinic:

- Euoquol 5D (Brazier et al. 1993), to assess functional status;
- the Hospital Anxiety and Depression scale (HAD) (Zigmond and Snaith 1983), to assess emotional disorder function.

Information from this pilot found that patients' outcomes locally were found to be similar as reported by other studies of critical care survivors (Eddleston and White 2000; Jones and Griffiths 1994; Jones et al. 1998). The Euroquol 5D indicated that 71% of patients attending these clinics had an overall reduced quality of life at three months post discharge from ITU, when matched to the general population for age and gender. The main clinical symptoms patients were found to have:

- weight loss
- reduced muscle strength
- fatigue
- functional/mobility difficulties
- difficulty sleeping
- delusional memory/nightmares
- little or no recall of the stay in ICU.

Using the HAD scale it was shown that 18% of patients had borderline levels of anxiety and 10% had borderline levels of depression. As informative for clinical practice, however, were the personal reports patients and their families described as the individual experience of their time in hospital. Many patients and families reported in feedback evaluating the clinics that simply by attending and having time to talk through their time in intensive care had helped them greatly. They appreciated an explanation for both physical and psychological symptoms they had been experiencing. They also informed us that this type of information would have been useful before leaving hospital. By amalgamating all of these results, the nursing staff running the clinic created a picture of what could have been improved upon during the patients' hospital stay. Combining the quantitative data and the qualitative information we were able to examine the areas of the patients' care pathway that required improvement.

From this short pilot the following have been introduced to improve the care pathway for the patients and their families:

- an information leaflet when patients are transferred to the ward;
- rehabilitation exercises devised for the individual patient by the physiotherapists;
- an audit of nutritional standards in intensive care;
- planned introduction of patient diaries.

While a formal follow-up clinic is the most advantageous method of assessing intensive care patients, in 2002 only 34% of hospitals had such a service (DoH 2003). As previously described there are difficulties in funding a clinic which potentially can cost £30,000 per year. The advantage of running a pilot clinic demonstrated for local requirements we needed a follow-up service for patients that started in the intensive care unit, through to discharge, as suggested in Critical to Success (Audit Commission 1999). We established that for the majority of patients who have been admitted/ventilated for less than 48 hours, follow-up in a formal clinic is not necessary; however, these patients still need to be assessed individually by critical care outreach for individual needs. Using this process patients who may need more formal follow-up can be identified, ensuring any clinic time is utilised fully; however, this does rely on the critical care outreach nurse being able to monitor patients for longer, within the constraints of their workload.

CRITICAL CARE OUTREACH: THE VITAL LINK FOR FOLLOW-UP IN THE GENERAL WARDS

The outreach nurses are therefore essential in ensuring that rehabilitation of intensive care patients continues in the ward areas. It enhances their role as the communicators between intensive care and the general wards, ensuring the care pathway for intensive care patients to discharge is seamless. Part of this will be acting as the advocates of the patients and their families, to influence care given in the general wards. Outreach nurses also need to act as educators and communicators to ward staff and other members of the multidisciplinary team. Staff in general wards are usually unaware of the physical and psychological effects a stay in intensive care can cause. Part of the educational programmes for ward staff needs to inform them of this, and so understand the reasons for some patients' slow progress, as well as managing patients in the acute phase of illness. Some patients who have had a long stay in intensive care may require time for explanations of the care they received, and an understanding of physical and psychological issues that may be affecting them. Critical care outreach nurses also need to feed back to the critical care units any clinical and operational issues they find when following up patients in the ward areas. Such a feedback mechanism can stimulate debate to improve patient care along the care pathway.

The extent to which the outreach nurse can influence the follow-up aspect of the role will depend in part on the size of the team, and the human resource available. The *National Outreach Report* (DoH 2003) showed that the delivery of critical care outreach varies considerably across the country. Some trusts do not yet have any sort of outreach service, while others vary from the lone nurse consultant, and only 25% of trusts offer a 24-hour seven-day a week service. Clearly the amount of time that can be devoted to ensuring the physical and psychological rehabilitation of intensive care patients will depend on the time available in the outreach team. There are many expectations on the critical care outreach team as shown in Figure 8.1. Nurses in the critical care outreach team need to maintain links, and clinical skills in the critical care units, to enhance the relationship and ensure communication between the two areas. They are required to maintain knowledge of clinical and service developments in the clinical area, and so enable the integration of any requirements for follow-up of patients. The need to manage all of these components indicates that a critical care outreach nurse requires the following skills to manage the follow-up of patients on the wards:

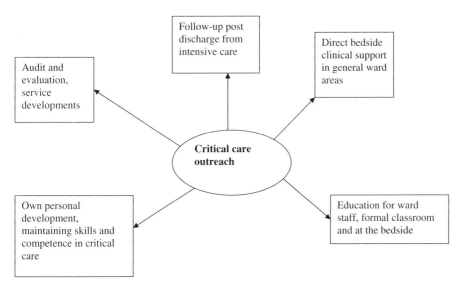

Figure 8.1 The multi-components of a critical care outreach service.

- clinical knowledge and expertise in critical care;
- a knowledge and understanding of the long-term physical and psychological effects of admission to critical care;
- communication skills;
- ability and autonomy to refer to other members of the multi-disciplinary team for further rehabilitation.

Conclusion

'When there is no data about subsequent quality of life, there is no evidence on which to base decisions about improvements to the practice of critical care, except in terms of what affects survival' (Audit Commission 1999). The challenge to critical care outreach is to ensure that as well as the acute phase of illness, patients are monitored for long-term follow-up in ward areas prior to discharge from hospital. This way critical care outreach nurses can ensure by working with and acting as the link between intensive care and the ward teams that the patient journey is enhanced by the knowledge and expertise of the specialist nurse. The importance of the whole in patient experience, evidence-based and tailored to the individual to promote independence is the next phase of the modernisation of the health service (DoH 2004b). To enable and maintain this part of the service, critical care outreach need to ensure these aspects are highlighted in business cases for future funding of the service.

REFERENCES

Angus DC, Carlet J (2003) Surviving intensive care: a report from the 2002 Brussels Roundtable. *Intensive Care Medicine* 29: 368–77.

Association of Anaesthetists (1988) *Intensive Care Services, Provision for the Future.* London: AAGBI.

Audit Commission (1999) Critical to success. *The Place of Efficient and Effective Critical Care Services within the Acute Hospital.* London: Audit Commission, October 1999.

Bion J, Heffner JE (2004) Challenges in the care of the acutely ill. *Lancet* 363: 970–8.

Brazier J, Jones N, Kind P (1993) Testing the validity of the Euroquol and comparing it with the SF 36 health survey questionnaire. *Quality of Life Research* 2: 169–80.

Crocker C (2003) A multidisciplinary follow-up clinic after patients' discharge from ITU. *British Journal of Nursing* 12(15): 910–14.

Department of Health (2000) *Comprehensive Critical Care: A Review of Adult Critical Care Services.* London: HMSO.

Department of Health (2003) *Progress in Developing Services: The National Outreach Report.* London: HMSO.

Department of Health (2004a) *10 High Impact Changes for Service Improvement and Delivery.* London: HMSO.

Department of Health (2004b) *National Standards, Local Action: Health and Social Care Standards and Planning Framework 2005/6–2007/08*. London: HMSO.

Eddleston J, White P (2000) Survival, morbidity, and quality of life after discharge from intensive care. *Critical Care Medicine* 28(7): 2293–9.

Gardner A, Sibthorpe B (2002) Will he get back to normal? Survival and functional status after intensive care therapy. *Intensive and Critical Care Nursing* 18: 138–45.

Goldfrad C, Rowan K (2000) Consequences of discharges from intensive care at night. *Lancet* 355, 1138–42.

Goldhill DR, Sumner A (1998) Outcome of intensive care patients in a group of British intensive care units. *Critical Care Medicine* 26(8): 1337–45.

Griffiths RD, Jones C (2002) *Intensive Care Aftercare*. Oxford: Butterworth-Heinemann.

Hayes JA, Black NA (2000) Outcome measures for adult critical care: a systematic review. *Health Technology Assessment* 4(24).

Johnson P, Chaboyer W, Foster M, Van Der Vooren R (2001) Care givers of ICU patients discharged home: What burden do they face? *Intensive and Critical Care Nursing* 17: 219–27.

Jones C, Griffiths RD (1994) Psychological problems occurring after intensive care. *British Journal of Intensive Care* February, 46–50.

Jones C, Humphris G, Griffiths RD (1998) Psychological morbidity following critical illness – the rationale for care after intensive care. *Clinical Intensive Care* 9: 199–205.

Jones C, Griffiths RD, Humphris G, Skirrow PM (2001) Memory, delusions, and the development of acute post traumatic stress disorder related symptoms after intensive care. *Critical Care Medicine* 29(3): 573–80.

Jones C, Skirrow P, Griffiths RD et al. (2003) Rehabilitation after critical illness: A randomised controlled trial. *Critical Care Medicine* 31(10): 2456–61.

Keenan SP, Dodek P, Chan K, Simon M, Hogg RS, Anis AH et al. (2004) Intensive care unit survivors have fewer hospital readmissions and readmission days than other hospitalized patients in British Columbia. *Critical Care Medicine* 32(2): 391–8.

McGloin H, Adam S, Singer M (1997) The quality of pre-ICU care, influences outcome of patients admitted from the ward. *Clinical Intensive Care* 8: 104.

McQuillan P, Pilkington S, Allan A et al. (1998) Confidential inquiry into quality of care before admission to intensive care. *British Medical Journal* 316: 1853–8.

Metcalf A, McPherson K (1995) *Study of the Provision of Intensive Care in England, 1993: Revised Report for the Department of Health*, London School of Hygiene and Tropical Medicine.

Ridley S (2002) Functional outcome after critical illness. *Care of the Critically Ill* 18(2): 44–7.

Sheffield Teaching Hospitals NHS Trust (2003) A follow up clinic service for intensive care patients: Results of a pilot study. Unpublished data. Sheffield.

Skirrow P, Jones C, Griffitths R, Kaney S (2001) Intensive care: easing the trauma. *The Psychologist* 14(12): 640–2.

Zigmond AS, Snaith RP (1983) The hospital anxiety and depression scale. *Acta Psychiatrica Scandinavica* 67: 361–70.

9 Patient diaries

WAYNE ROBSON, GAYLE WHEELDON AND
DENISE PENNEY

Critical care outreach nurses can spend a significant part of their time follow-ing up patients who have been on intensive care. Some of these patients remember very little about their stay; others have some factual memories along with delusional memories (Jones et al. 2001). This amnesia can make it hard for patients to appreciate how ill they have actually been and why they are now feeling tired and weak.

During follow-up visits to the ward the outreach nurse often fills in any gaps in the patient's memory and may discuss any frightening or delusional memories that the patient may have experienced. To try and help patients make sense of their time in ICU, some units in the 1990s began keeping diaries for patients which also included photographs of the patient while they were sedated and attached to a ventilator. This chapter will discuss the need for patient diaries and review studies that have tried to evaluate whether they offer any benefit to patients recovering from a stay on ICU. The chapter will also share the experiences of Chesterfield Royal Hospital ICU in establishing patient diaries, providing an insight into some of the challenges and potential obstacles for others interested in introducing this initiative. The following points will be addressed in the chapter.

- What is an ICU patient diary?
- Why is there a need for patient diaries?
- Is there any evidence that patient diaries help recovery from ICU? A brief review of the literature.
- Introducing patient diaries into practice: The experiences of a district general hospital.

WHAT EXACTLY IS AN ICU PATIENT DIARY?

As the name suggests, a patient diary is a small (A5 size) notebook (see Figure 9.1) which is kept by the patient's bedside and is an ongoing account

Critical Care Outreach. Edited by Lee Cutler and Wayne Robson.
Copyright 2006 by John Wiley & Sons Ltd.

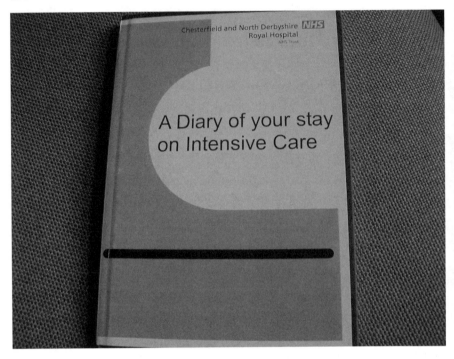

Chesterfield and North Derbyshire **NHS**
Royal Hospital
NHS Trust

A Diary of your stay
on Intensive Care

Figure 9.1

of activities and events that have happened to the patient during their stay in
ICU. Photographs will also be taken of the patient at various stages of their
illness, for example when they were sedated and attached to a ventilator or
haemofiltration machine, and these are later included in the diary if the
patient wishes to have them. Nursing staff usually make entries in the diaries
each day. Friends and relatives are also encouraged to write in the diaries so
that patients have an account of events happening within their day-to-day
lives as individuals. For some family members the diary provides an opportunity to express their feelings about the patient in a way that they may find
difficult to communicate to a patient who is sedated and unable to respond.

Diaries are considered for all patients who are expected to stay on ICU for
more than four or five days, and the diary builds an account of the circumstances of their admission, and the time they have 'lost' while sedated.

The text in the diary is written in 'layman's' terms avoiding medical jargon
or anything that might break confidentiality. Staff often relay words of encouragement and provide simple explanations of different procedures that the
patient may have been through. Nurses and other staff groups are advised
only to include information that they would be comfortable relaying verbally

to the patient or relatives at the bedside. Box 9.1 provides some examples of the kind of entries that are commonly found in patient diaries.

Box 9.1 Examples of entries in patient diaries

Hello . . . . , my name is Wayne and I am one of the nurses. We are writing this diary to help you understand the time you spent with us on intensive care. You were brought to the A&E department on Wednesday, 3rd September after falling from a ladder while you were cleaning your windows. You have broken your pelvis and seven of your ribs. You also have a head injury and there is some swelling of your brain . . .

Hello . . . . , my name is Francis and I am the nurse looking after you on the night shift. We have had a quiet night and I cannot believe how much you have improved since I last looked after you a week ago. You are now breathing on your own without the ventilator, but you are still needing some drugs to keep your blood pressure at a normal level . . .

All groups of staff who come into contact with the patient are encouraged to make entries – nurses, doctors and physiotherapists – thereby affording the patient a good overall picture of their stay. Patient diaries and photographs are only shown to patients once they have left ICU and are recovering, and then only if the patient wishes to see them.

WHY IS THERE A NEED FOR PATIENT DIARIES?

Being critically ill on ICU can be a very traumatic experience, indeed it is estimated that up to 27% of this group of patients can experience post-traumatic stress disorder (PTSD) (Schelling et al. 1998). This disorder is characterised by intrusive memories of the traumatic event, avoidance of things associated with the event, and symptoms of arousal (American Psychiatric Association 1994).

Having delusional memories, but no factual memories, of a stay in ICU is thought to be associated with an increased risk of developing PTSD. Jones et al. (2001) examined the relationship between memories of ICU and the development of PTSD related symptoms in a group of 45 patients discharged from ICU. Patients with delusional memories but no factual recall of ICU scored highly when tested for PTSD related symptoms. The authors concluded that factual memories of real events, even if they were relatively unpleasant, may provide some protection from anxiety, and from the development of PTSD related symptoms in patients with delusional memories. The factual information may help the patient challenge the delusional memories. Jones et al. (2001) suggest:

> A frightening memory of a nurse trying to kill you without a balancing memory of care received in the ICU is likely to have great importance and emotional significance to the patient. (p. 576)

It also appears that in other types of traumatic life experiences factual information can help patients make sense of memories or events. Kinsler (1990) describes a child survivor of the Holocaust who continually had flashbacks of trains, but did not know why. She thought she was going crazy, until one day in a meeting of survivors someone explained that at the place where she had stayed trains could be seen through the bars of the children's barracks. She was relieved to discover that she was not going crazy.

Patient diaries might be one way of providing patients with factual information about their time in ICU, and as in the above example this may help them understand any strange or disturbing memories or flashbacks.

The amnesia that some patients experience about their time on ICU may affect not only their own psychological well-being but also that of their relatives. Young et al. (2005) found that relatives of ICU patients had a significantly higher number of symptoms of anxiety than the ICU patients themselves at three months post-discharge. Young et al. (2005) hypothesised that the patients' amnesia may contribute to this finding by causing a lack of shared memory/understanding between patients and relatives, which then presents a psychological burden to relatives.

Other studies have also highlighted that post-ICU, patients have a strong need to understand what has happened to them. McKinney and Deeny (2002) interviewed patients who had transferred from ICU to a general ward, and one of the themes identified from the data was 'restoring meaning'. Patients were keen to revisit their experience cognitively in order to restore some meaning and make sense of what has happened to them. Compton (1991) revealed that patients found a lack of information about their stay in ICU very frustrating and that some of them spent a lot of effort trying to piece events together. This was mainly done by asking friends and relatives to fill in the gaps in their memories. This suggests that there is a significant demand for initiatives like the diaries among post-ICU patients to help them make sense of their critical illness.

IS THERE ANY EVIDENCE THAT DIARIES HELP RECOVERY FROM ICU? A BRIEF REVIEW OF THE LITERATURE

Using patient diaries for unconscious patients appears to have originated as an idea in Denmark in 1984 (Nordvedt 1987). Patient diaries in ICU appear to have developed mostly in Sweden where a number of small studies have been carried out to try to evaluate the use of the diaries. Probably the largest of these evaluations was that carried out by Backman and Walther (2001).

Backman and Walther (2001) carried out a questionnaire study to evaluate the usefulness of patient diaries. The sample comprised 41 patients who had accepted a diary and 10 relatives of non-survivors who had accepted their loved ones' diary. Questionnaires were sent to patients six months after their discharge.

All respondents stated that they had shared their diary with relatives and friends, and felt that it had helped them understand their time on ICU. Twenty-six of the diaries had been read more than ten times and comments made in the questionnaires were mostly positive or very positive, and this also included comments from bereaved relatives.

Since the early 2000s there has been growing interest in ICU diaries in the UK, although very little to date has been published about the UK experiences.

Combe (2005) describes the introduction of patient diaries into an ICU in the UK following findings from their follow-up clinic that indicated that patients had poor recollections of their time on ICU, and were troubled by the gaps in their memory.

Feedback from patients who had been given diaries was positive. They found the photographs helped them appreciate how sick they had been. Bereaved relatives also found the diaries helpful in that: 'they had some concrete memory of their loved ones' last days before they died' (p. 34).

Diaries also appear to have been used in other areas outside adult general ICUs. A similar approach for example has been used in neonatal intensive care. Stenson (1996) describes the use of patient diaries in this setting. Nursing staff write letters to the parents from the baby, describing what is happening from the baby's viewpoint. Stenson (1996) describes how the diaries help promote attachment and 'generate positive memories' (p. 1615). The diaries have been positively received and copies of the diaries have also been given to bereaved parents.

Journal writing or diaries also seem to have been used to encourage patients to disclose their experiences of a traumatic event through entries in a diary or journal.

Barry and Singer (2001) demonstrated that mothers who had experienced having a child admitted to the neonatal intensive care unit had reduced psychological stress after the event if they wrote about their experiences in a journal each day for four days. It may be possible that the relatives of adult ICU patients who make entries in their loved one's diary may also gain some similar kind of psychological benefit. Anecdotally, relatives of patients from Chesterfield Royal Hospital ICU have commented that they found writing in their loved one's diary gave them something to focus upon and helped them feel they were doing something positive for the patient.

INTRODUCING PATIENT DIARIES: THE EXPERIENCES OF A DISTRICT GENERAL HOSPITAL

Chesterfield Royal Hospital in Derbyshire, UK, introduced patient diaries into their ICU in October 2003. The following is an account of the implementation process and some of the challenges and barriers that were faced.

THE IMPLEMENTATION PROCESS

Prior to the introduction of the diaries, articles about the use of patient diaries in Sweden were made available for all staff to read. A small group of interested staff was formed, and the group visited another hospital in the UK (Whiston Hospital, Merseyside) that had already introduced the diaries. A comprehensive guideline for how patient diaries would operate was then written. Advice was sought from the patient safety team regarding issues of consent to start a diary and take photographs of sedated patients. Funding was secured to buy stocks of hardback diary notebooks, and a digital camera with stocks of photographic paper. Teaching sessions were delivered to all staff and a launch date was set.

CHALLENGES AND CONCERNS

Taking photographs of patients when they cannot consent

Many staff expressed concerns about the ethics of taking a patient's photograph when they were sedated and could not consent. The relatives give their approval to take a photograph, and the photograph is then stored securely in a locked cabinet. The patient will be given the opportunity to see the photograph when they have recovered.

The photograph can be saved if the patient is unsure about looking at it at that time in their recovery, or alternatively the photograph can be destroyed if the patient wishes.

Photographs are taken sensitively, not too close up and in a way that shows the equipment that the patient was attached to. The justification for taking the photograph is that this is done with the patients' best interests in mind, to give them a choice of being able to see the photos if they wish, something which is thought to help them in their recovery. Published evaluations of patient diaries indicate that patients do want to look at and keep their photographs, and our experiences at Chesterfield support this.

Finding the time to make entries in the diaries

For nurses and other health professionals, time is a precious resource, and there seems to be increasingly more tasks and documentation to complete.

Maintaining patient diaries in this culture can be difficult. Nurses from ICU need to be encouraged to take part in the handover of diaries when patients have recovered so that they can see the potential benefits to the patient of trying to spend a few minutes every day making entries in the diaries. However, releasing nurses from ICU to hand diaries over to patients can be another additional challenge as many units are constantly busy.

What happens to the diary if the patient dies on ICU?

Up to 25% of patients on ICU do not survive, and therefore there will always be a number of patients who die while their diaries are in progress or die after leaving ICU before the diary has been handed over to them. In this scenario relatives are contacted to ask if they would like to have their loved ones' diary and photographs. Our experience from Chesterfield Royal Hospital has been that most relatives do wish to have the diary and photographs, and appear to find it some comfort. Published evaluations of the use of patient diaries also support our experiences (Backman and Walther 2001; Combe 2005).

Critical care outreach nurses are in an excellent position to be involved with patient diaries. They can make an entry in the diary before the patient leaves ICU, introducing themselves and explaining how they will be visiting the patient on the general ward. They are also very well placed to liaise with staff from ICU and the wards to identify if and when the patient is ready to look at their diary.

Patient diaries are a simple and inexpensive way of helping patients understand the time they spent on ICU. The process of helping to construct the diary may be helpful and even cathartic for relatives. Further research is required to evaluate patients' and relatives' experiences of the diaries.

ACKNOWLEDGEMENTS

The authors would like to acknowledge the help and support of Dr Christina Jones from Whiston Hospital ICU when they were establishing patient diaries at Chesterfield Royal Hospital intensive care unit.

REFERENCES

American Psychiatric Association (1994) *Diagnostic and Statistical Manual of Mental Disorders* 4th edn. Washington DC.

Backman CG, Walther SM (2001) Use of a personal diary written on the ICU during critical illness. *Intensive Care Medicine* 27: 426–9.

Barry LM, Singer GH (2001) Reducing maternal psychological distress after the NICU experience, through journal writing. *Journal of Early Intervention* 24(4): 287–97.

Combe D (2005) The use of patient diaries in an intensive care unit. *Nursing in Critical Care* 10(1): 31–4.

Compton P (1991) Critical illness and intensive care: what it means to the client. *Critical Care Nursing* 11: 50–6.

Jones C, Griffiths RD, Humphris G, Skirrow P (2001) Memory, delusions, and the development of acute post traumatic stress disorder-related symptoms after intensive care. *Critical Care Medicine* 29(3): 573–80.

Kinsler F (1990) The dynamics of brief group therapy in homogenous populations: Child survivors of the holocaust. Paper presented for the Sixth Annual Meeting of the International Society for Traumatic Stress Studies. New Orleans.

McKinney A A, Deeny P (2002) Leaving the intensive care unit: a phenomenological study of the patients' experience. *Intensive and Critical Care Nursing* 18: 320–31.

Nordvedt L (1987) Dialog i sykepleie [Dialogue in nursing]. *Sykepleien* 74(20): 6–11.

Schelling G, Stoll C, Meier M (1998) Health related quality of life and post traumatic stress disorder in survivors of adult respiratory distress syndrome. *Critical Care Medicine* 26: 651–9.

Stenson B (1996) Promoting attachment, providing memories. *British Medical Journal* 313: 1651.

Young E, Eddleston J, Ingleby S et al. (2005) Returning home after intensive care: a comparison of symptoms of anxiety and depression in ICU and elective cardiac surgery patients and their relatives. *Intensive Care Medicine* 31: 86–91.

IV Managing and Supporting Outreach Practitioners

10 Establishing and managing a critical care outreach team: a practical approach

ALEX LARKIN

INTRODUCTION

Current government policy and modernisation in healthcare delivery are inextricably linked with the development of a workforce that has flexible teams, working to 'expand and cross professional and organisational boundaries' (DoH 2000a, 2001). This approach to workforce development attempts to ensure that all staff are enabled to make the best use of their skills, knowledge and competencies in order to place the patient effectively at the centre of health care delivery (DoH 1999, 2000a, 2000c). The development of a new critical care outreach service presented an ideal opportunity to capitalise on the concept of multi-professional, cross-boundary team working. This innovative model of service delivery was new to the critical care team in the author's hospital, and presented some key challenges and opportunities around a wide range of issues, including recruiting and building a team, integration of the team into existing services, supporting and developing the team and monitoring and improving standards and services.

Distilled from real life experience, this chapter uses both theoretical and empirical knowledge to illustrate the author's experiences in practice, and provides a rationale for the strategies employed. It aims to present the reader with a description of the key themes and challenges encountered, illustrate the approaches used and identify the lessons learned in the establishment and management of a critical care outreach team.

BACKGROUND

Formed in April 2002, the Pennine Acute Hospitals NHS Trust is a merged trust employing 10,000 staff across five hospital sites, including:

Critical Care Outreach. Edited by Lee Cutler and Wayne Robson.
Copyright 2006 by John Wiley & Sons Ltd.

- Fairfield General Hospital, Bury
- North Manchester General Hospital
- The Royal Oldham Hospital
- Rochdale Infirmary
- Birch Hill Hospital, Rochdale.

The merger resulted in the formation of one of the largest non-teaching hospitals in the United Kingdom, serving a population of approximately 800,000.

In late 1999 (prior to the merger), the trust board were asked to consider a business case for the development of an 'at risk assessor' whose primary role would be to enhance the recognition and management of acutely unwell patients, thereby improving their experience and outcomes.

The publication of *Comprehensive Critical Care* (DoH 2000d) combined with this preliminary work to convince the former Oldham NHS Trust to bid successfully for ring-fenced outreach development monies.

In April 2001, I was appointed to the post of consultant nurse in critical care. The main remit for this post was to:

> be an expert clinically based practitioner who will strengthen the nursing contri-
> bution to critically ill patients cared for across the hospital. A key priority for the
> post holder will be to develop and implement a patient at risk scoring system for
> use in acute clinical areas.

In collaboration with clinical colleagues, the trust board and the hospital critical care steering group, and taking account of Department of Health guidance, key service objectives were defined and an operational policy was devised. This policy retained enough flexibility to ensure that the detail of the delivery of the service could be decided locally (Ovretveit 1997). The development of a clear operational policy also enabled us to consider what the outreach service would not do (see Box 10.1).

Box 10.1 Outreach service objectives and what outreach will not do

Outreach service objectives:

- to identify patients at risk of clinical deterioration and provide timely intervention, averting admission to critical care where possible
- to assist with the management plan and treatment of critically

Outreach will not:

- provide a stop gap for staff shortages
- treat and transfer all critically ill patients
- attend all cardiac arrests
- be used to fulfil the role of junior doctors

ill patients on the ward, and facilitate their admission to level 2/3 care if necessary
- to enable discharges from the critical care area
- to assess and meet the educational needs of staff caring for level 1–3 patients
- to share critical care skills with ward staff

- de-skill ward staff and parent teams
- disempower ward staff and parent teams
- diminish ward staff roles
- promote over-reliance on the outreach team

RECRUITMENT OF THE OUTREACH TEAM

Box 10. 2 Recruitment of the outreach team

The main challenges identified include:

- recruiting and developing an effective multi-professional team to a new service – promoting new ways of working;
- ensuring the correct skill mix within the team;
- establishing each team member's ability to work independently and collaboratively.

The formation of the new outreach service presented an opportunity for a creative approach to recruitment. A number of policy initiatives have set the scene for creative and new ways of working (DoH 1999, 2000c). This modern concept must be actively fostered so that it becomes integrated into the culture of the organisation (Kenny 2002).

Effective teams facilitate the development of shared beliefs, values, goals and vision, both within and among clinical teams (Kenny 2002). Teams must also be able to function on an inter-professional and multi-professional basis, that is, as a group of different professionals they are required to come together and work within the team, and they are also required to work on a multi-professional basis with other healthcare providers outside of the team (Scholes and Vaughan 2002).

Definition of a team:

A group of people (different professionals) assembling to achieve a common goal. (Ovretveit 1997)

The job descriptions were developed with an emphasis on the need for competent and experienced practitioners. An advanced level of clinical knowledge, decision-making and communication skills were of paramount importance. There would be a requirement for the post holders to step out of their comfort zone, often working on their own. This demanded a high level of professional maturity and experiential wisdom. The service and operational policy required the appointment of a team that possessed the right blend of skills, knowledge and attitude to undertake the complex mix of activities required (see Figure 10.1). A multi-professional team was actively recruited in order to enhance the success of the service (DoH 2000a; Hill and Ingala 2001).

In November 2001, three full-time staff were appointed to the post of outreach practitioner: a senior 1 physiotherapist with critical care experience and two senior nurses, one with intensive care experience and one with high dependency care experience. Though each individual brings their own unique strengths to the role, each practitioner operates to the same job description. A senior critical care nurse was also appointed to the post of practice based educator.

In March 2003, an associate specialist was appointed to provide eight clinical sessions per week for outreach, combined with clinical sessions on the critical care units.

Clerical support is provided on a part-time basis. This has proved to be invaluable in terms of capturing relevant audit data, producing reports and providing administrative support to all members of the team.

This mix of clinicians and support staff has provided the service with an incredibly broad range of advanced competencies that serve to meet the needs of the organisation, staff groups and the patient in a flexible manner (see Table 10.1).

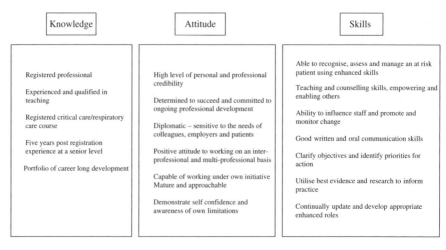

Figure 10.1 Identified skills, knowledge and attitude for the critical care outreach practitioner.

Table 10.1 Range of competencies possessed by critical care outreach practitioners

Team competencies that meet organisational needs	Team competencies that meet staff needs	Team competencies that meet patient needs
• Knowledge and understanding of the complex healthcare system • Appropriate use of scarce critical care resources • Management of risk and support for the clinical governance agenda • Development of services to improve patient care • Delivery of a flexible and responsive service • Audit and data collection to inform services and resource issues	• Expert clinical advice • Educational provision for the multi-professional teams in acute clinical areas • Working collaboratively • Implementing evidence based practice • Practical support in delivery of care when required • Enhanced clinical roles • Support pre and post registration clinical placements for nurses and doctors • Empowered and enabled to deliver enhanced care • Staff and career development – role model	• Deliver and coordinate elements of care for the whole patient journey • Supporting the delivery of the right care, in the right place by the right person/team • Acting as the patient advocate • Delivery of expert clinical practice • Improving experience and outcomes • Preventing adverse incidents

The benefits of team working and the pooling of unique professional knowledge, experience and expertise are supported by a growing evidence base (Cook et al. 2001). Combining the collective competencies of the team and sharing individual skills and knowledge have ensured that the service has evolved to be one that is patient focused, considering all aspects of the patient journey. The contribution that other professional groups make is acknowledged and valued. There are also benefits in terms of career progression for others as they see the practitioners as credible role models, generating new ways of working from their own professional sphere, without losing their professional identity (DoH 2000a).

Box 10. 3 Lessons learned/tips to ensure success

• Don't assume all other staff groups will embrace a multi-professional approach.
• Awareness raising about new ways of working within and outside of the team is helpful.
• Consider 'team' competencies rather than individual competencies.
• Capitalise on each other's strengths and be honest about areas for development.
• Re-focusing professional identities and moving away from 'comfort zones' can take time.

MANAGING OUTREACH AND THE WIDER TEAM: DEVELOPING A SHARED VISION

Box 10.4

The main challenges identified include:

• developing a shared vision within and outside the team;
• gaining sponsorship from key groups of staff and the organisation;
• integrating a new service into established ways of working.

Critical care outreach was a new concept for the trust. It was important therefore to spend some time considering what the critical care outreach service would look like; what it would do and how it would achieve its objectives. In order to make this change in practice an enduring success, time and effort were invested in developing an understanding of the clinical environment in which the service would be delivered – a 'situational analysis' (Outhwaite 2003).

It is easy to attribute the failure of any new concept to the personalities of the individuals involved. While it is important to consider the individual, it is imperative that the change itself is carefully orchestrated in order to provide the right environment for success (Reay et al. 2003). Creating a shared vision among the multi-professional team and the organisation is essential to cultivating a sense of ownership of the service. This serves to incorporate the wider team into the outreach service and reinforces their role in fulfilling the objective of enhanced patient care (Williams 2004).

There was a need to gain sponsorship and support from the key groups of staff with whom the outreach team interact on a daily basis. This sponsorship and support were imperative if a successful shared vision was to truly exist. A large amount of time was therefore devoted to promoting the benefits of the outreach service. An effective strategy was to arrange meetings with key individuals in order to promote the service and gauge their likely response. Several divisional meetings were attended, some of which were uni-professional and some multi-professional. Educational sessions and progress updates were also undertaken. These sessions were designed to be interactive and provided valuable information about what was already 'out there', thus helping to prevent service duplication and professional 'jostling' for roles (Freeman et al. 2000).

A vast range of staff responses to the proposed service were voiced at these meetings, ranging from 'but we already do that, why do we need more specialist nurses to do the basics?' to 'what a fantastic idea – when do you start?'

Interestingly, it was the senior staff who were ambivalent towards the introduction of the service and defensive of their own clinical practice (Reay et al. 2003). In order to try and allay any fears or concerns, there was an emphasis upon weaving the outreach service into the current clinical teams and systems thus complementing the existing service, rather than being considered a disruption and additional burden. Staff were given the opportunity to discuss any concerns or issues, and awareness sessions took place to ensure that staff groups understood the need for the service and the change in practice (Outhwaite 2003).

Trust board and management sponsorship was maintained and mobilised by keeping the organisation informed with short presentations, and by updates at weekly board meetings via the executive nurse. Case studies proved to be a very powerful method of encouraging the organisation to 'buy into' the concept of outreach (Vincent et al. 2001):

Mrs X was an 83 year old lady, previously fit and well, admitted to the hospital with a 3 day history of diarrhoea, vomiting and a small amount of rectal bleeding. She deteriorated over the next 3 days in hospital and eventually was admitted to ITU where she died. A retrospective application of the early warning score highlighted the onset and development of her acute deterioration 24 hours after admission. The patient was not seen by a senior member of the team for a further 48 hours, resulting in a delay in diagnosis and late admission to ITU.

Case studies also serve to highlight the fact that clinical and organisational issues are intertwined. Focusing on only one aspect of health care, without understanding the processes involved, does a great disservice to the patient, the staff and the organisation (Risser et al. 1999).

It was decided that the most effective way of introducing the service would be to adopt a model based on a philosophy of empowering and enabling the clinical staff to recognise and care for acutely unwell patients, and to formulate and implement appropriate management plans. The operational policy was then developed and used to provide the framework within which the team is able to function in a consistent manner. This framework has been translated into team objectives and a shared vision, which influences service provision and a clear direction. Clarity of vision and purpose has enabled the team to build its own identity and carve out its professional boundaries (Outhwaite 2003).

Box 10.5 Lessons learned/tips to ensure success

- Take time to understand the clinical areas where the service will be introduced.
- Network and undertake public relations exercises to 'sell' the service.
- Look at things from the perspective of others.
- Introduce and manage the change in a structured manner.
- Don't be afraid to modify the original 'vision' in accordance with feedback from other members of staff.
- Address any issues promptly: minor problems may become major obstacles if not addressed immediately.
- Don't take resistance to change personally.

CREATIVE RESOURCE MANAGEMENT

Box 10.6

The main challenges identified include:

- providing an effective, high-quality service within limited resources;
- the need to change/influence the working practice of others without having managerial control.

One of the key issues to address was the lack of resources to provide a twenty-four-hour service; indeed the outreach team itself was a limited resource. In order to maximise the impact of the service, and to ensure integration into the clinical environment, the groups of staff already operating in the clinical areas – the wider team – must be acknowledged and understood. These staff groups are delivering care within the general clinical areas, though they may not necessarily be based within those areas (see Figure 10.2).

In focusing on the detail of the role of the wider team, we were able to identify the night nurse practitioners (NNPs) as being able to deliver the outreach service at night.

There was an acknowledgement that the NNPs had been 'doing outreach' for some time, although this aspect of their role was never formally identified. The divisional managers were extremely receptive to recognising this important aspect of their work and it was identified clearly as a distinct element of their job description.

This was advantageous in two ways. First, in combination with the night nurse practitioner service, the outreach team could ensure a seamless service, twenty-four hours a day, seven days a week. This consistent presence has ensured that the whole patient journey is monitored and contributed to. The team have developed a detailed knowledge about the systems that the patient is managed within, and this has enabled them to develop the ability to predict more accurately when gaps or discontinuities in care, in the system and in the service might contribute to a potential or actual adverse event for the patient. Having identified the potential problems, the team are able to take a proactive approach to bridge the gaps in care, resulting in a positive impact on patient

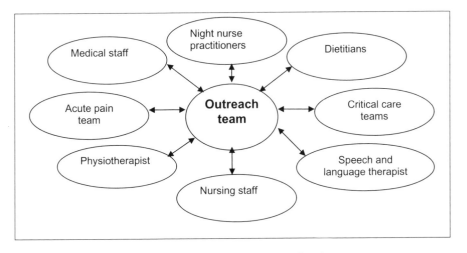

Figure 10.2 Wider 'team members'.

safety (Risser et al. 1999; Cook et al. 2000). Secondly the NNP role was enhanced, clinically enriched and more clearly defined.

The consultant nurse, senior NNP manager and indeed the team members, have worked collaboratively in order to promote a shared vision and work in synergy towards common goals. A number of initiatives have helped to bring this about.

1. As far as possible, working practices for outreach service delivery are shared.
2. An explicit understanding of the goals of outreach exists and serves to influence the practice on night duty.
3. Joint training sessions are held and 'face-to-face' handovers take place at the beginning and end of each shift.

This collaborative approach has exploited opportunities to enhance and improve patient care. Close liaison between the consultant nurse and the senior NNP ensures that the outreach service is effective and consistent twenty-four hours per day.

Multi-professional members of the wider team also work collaboratively with the outreach service in order to ensure that the patient needs are met in a timely manner. A large number of referrals are both made and received from a wide group of staff (see Figure 10.3).

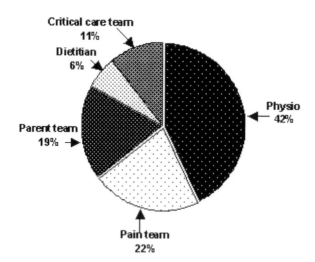

Figure 10.3 Referrals by outreach to other members of the multi-professional team.

This frequency of multi-professional interaction is testament to the belief that outreach cannot operate in a vacuum and is everyone's business. It also illustrates the complex nature of acutely unwell patients, the cooperative nature of the service delivered, and the value placed on the contribution of others.

Box 10.7 Lessons learned and tips for success

- Promote the benefits of changing practice as a 'win–win' issue.
- Provide compelling evidence about the need to change.
- Understand and acknowledge the workload and resource issues of other teams.
- Understand and acknowledge the contribution of others to the overall success of the outreach service.
- Introduce change using small steps and review the impact of each change.
- Share benefits as well as work, e.g. shared education sessions.
- Ensure regular face-to-face contact with other team members/professional colleagues.

LEADERSHIP

Box 10.8

Main challenges identified include:

- developing an appropriate leadership style;
- leading those for whom one has no managerial authority;
- motivating others to lead and develop.

The operational policy outlined the organisational aspects of the service: who does what, when and to whom. The leadership role is about setting the direction of travel and the means by which we will achieve our common goals: 'how do we do it?' (Ovretveit 1997).

To ensure that the operational goals are met, the team leader cultivates the development of a shared team vision, open communication, collaboration, mutual respect and equality (Freeman et al. 2000; Scholes and Vaughan 2002). In order for effective inter-professional team working to take place, professional socialisation is essential (Risser et al. 1999). Regular team discussions take place regarding clinical practice and service provision and development, aided by the fact that we all share one office! This can be highly distracting at times, but the benefits far outweigh any disadvantages. Close proximity has created the optimal physical environment in which to develop the team by promoting effective working relationships.

Equally as important, is the development of an appropriate organisational culture that embraces change and supports, promotes and implements ideas and creative thinking; a culture of 'care' (Truman 2000; Sheridan 2003b):

> the responsibility of a leader is to create the conditions to release potential energy. (Outhwaite 2003)

The transformational leadership role focuses on enabling individuals to best apply their skills, knowledge and efforts (Sheridan 2003b). All team members are involved in any service review or development. Following discussion and evaluation, the team members' suggestions are often the catalyst for change and have helped to ensure the service is fully responsive to the needs of all of its users (Simons 2003). Asking the team to propose suggestions for change and solutions as to how this can be achieved engenders a culture of responsibility. Implementing these ideas promotes ownership and is highly motivational (Hyrkas and Appelqvist-Schmidlechner 2003).

The team identified that patient care would be enhanced if they were able to order chest X rays and prescribe intravenous fluids. Protocols were developed and agreed by the trust, and training was delivered. While these developments have enhanced patient care, inadvertently they have also assisted other members of the clinical team.

Each team member is encouraged to take the lead on a project that is aligned to their specialist area of interest and expertise, thus fulfilling their requirements for professional development, while meeting the needs of the service. All contributions and successes, no matter how big or small, are acknowledged and attributed to the individual concerned. This approach ensures that the strengths of the individual are exposed, providing a net team profit (Belbin 1999).

Box 10.9 Lessons learned and tips for success

- Develop an appropriate leadership style – one size does not fit all!
- Be visible and accessible.
- Encourage radical thinking and promote a change culture.
- 'Stage manage' any changes in practice.
- Acknowledge the contribution of others – if something is another team member's idea, this must be recognised.

STAFF APPRAISAL, DEVELOPMENT AND CLINICAL SUPERVISION

Box 10.10

The main challenges identified include:

- ensuring quality of service provision;
- maintaining staff enthusiasm and promoting retention;
- all team members from a variety of backgrounds – staff development needs are very different;
- learning from adverse events.

Staff appraisal is a useful vehicle to promote quality of service delivery and enhance professional development. A strong association has been identified between the utilisation of appraisal tools and mortality rates (Morey et al. 2002). Investment in the ongoing development of skills and competencies is essential to ensuring quality, adds value to the service and supports recruitment, retention and the development of career pathways (DoH 2001; McKinley 2001). For the team leader, undertaking appraisals provides the opportunity to take a 'helicopter view' of the service and the individual team members, and permits the identification of common themes and problems that may need to be resolved.

Although the team were highly experienced and competent in their own fields, it was recognised that there were some educational issues that needed to be resolved (DoH 2001). There is a need to acknowledge each other's professional abilities, while also accepting that, if we were all to operate to the same job description, any gaps in our own knowledge and skills must be addressed. Regular teaching sessions are organised in response to clinical developments and the needs identified in the professional development plans.

Conflict and tensions may arise within the team, or between the team and other professional or managerial groups, and are often the result of challenging the status quo (Outhwaite 2003; Sheridan 2003a). It is important to understand the origin of the conflict and to work collaboratively to achieve patient-driven solutions to resolve them. Two-way communication that is open and honest is used to avoid or resolve conflict. There is an improved dialogue with previously isolated groups of professionals, e.g. dieticians, speech and language therapists, and a team member attends relevant forums for other groups with whom we interact, e.g. senior sisters meeting, junior doctor inductions.

Informal clinical supervision is used to identify and address any issues that need to be resolved and has proved to be a useful tool to deal with frustrations and aid development. Formal clinical supervision is encouraged if the individual feels that this would be beneficial. Team values and vision are clearly articulated and understood, which has aided the development of some ground rules and helped to establish mutual trust and professional respect:

• respect colleagues, patients and relatives;
• behave in a professional manner;
• value the skills and knowledge of others;
• communicate effectively (Walton 1984; Sheridan 2003a).

Our philosophy is grounded in a patient-centred approach. Using reflective practice to study cases from clinical practice is a very effective learning tool that enhances staff awareness, supports shared learning and provides opportunities for staff to improve the quality of care delivered (DoH 2000a).

Example of a case for reflection

It was identified that the number of readmissions to critical care was increasing, and staff were keen to investigate this and propose solutions to improve care processes (Outhwaite 2003).

Box 10.11

Admission details:
Young female patient admitted to critical care for overnight ventilation following a laparotomy.
Management on critical care:
Extubated the following morning. Sedation score 3. Poor cough.
Tachycardic throughout admission – HR 100–130
Other vital signs stable
WCC increased to $18 \times 10\,g/l$.
Discharge details:
RR on extubation 19, increased to 33 at point of discharge. BP 180/70, HR 130, pyrexial.
On 1 l oxygen via nasal cannula, O_2 saturation 99.
Decision to discharge to ward, asked by outreach to send to HDU.
Events prior to readmission:
Became increasingly short of breath, very chesty, RR 40, poor cough, oxygen saturation 98 on 1 litre O_2. ABGS: Ph 7.51, PaO_2 8.7, $PaCO_2$ 4.2
FiO_2 increased to 40%, went on to CPAP. CXR: underinflated, patchy basal consolidation, pulmonary oedema. Readmitted to ITU 48 hours later

Points for reflection/comment:

- Should the patient have been discharged?
- Could we have done anything to prevent this readmission?
- What can we learn from this case?
- Do we need to change any practice to prevent this from happening again?

The case reflection resulted in a number of changes. All patients have their early warning score recorded and are reviewed by outreach prior to discharge. Where the score is 3 or more, the discharge is delayed until a further medical review has been sought. These actions have resulted in a reduction in the number of readmissions to ITU.

All staff will have differing needs in terms of their professional and personal development, which must be facilitated for the mutual benefit of staff and patients alike. Professional and service development depends upon effective learning, which occurs due to a variety of approaches, and is not simply the result of attending formal educational sessions. Reflective practice, clinical supervision and agreed development plans are excellent vehicles to achieve learning.

Box 10.12 Lessons learned/tips for success

- Ensure appraisal systems are in place and development plans are reviewed and updated.
- Learn from adverse and successful clinical events to make positive changes and improvements to services.
- Both individual and team development, and personal and professional enhancement are inextricably linked.
- Learning is enhanced through utilising a combination of a range of techniques.

AUTHORITY, ACCOUNTABILITY AND RESPONSIBILITY

Box 10.13

The main challenges identified include:

- ensuring staff from multi-professional backgrounds had a common understanding of role boundaries, autonomy and authority;
- managing staff from different professional backgrounds.

Key to achieving clinical governance is the identification of clear boundaries and guidance around professional autonomy, accountability and responsibility (Ridgway and Maxwell 2001). While the autonomous nature of the outreach practitioner role is recognised, it is essential that their practice is set within a framework of relevant policies and procedures, in order to ensure the safety of both the patient and the individual practitioner (Ovretveit 1997).

Responsibilities that can be attributed to the individual practitioner are clearly outlined in the job descriptions, which are kept under review in the light of service developments (Ridgway and Maxwell 2001). Clear objectives are set at appraisal, and tasks/roles are negotiated and delegated. In order for the practitioner to fulfil their role effectively, a level of authority must also be delegated so that decisions can be made (Spath 2004). This delegated responsibility promotes job satisfaction through empowerment (DoH 2000f).

Also explicit in the job description are the lines of accountability: to whom the individuals are answerable. The team are accountable to the consultant nurse. It was thought initially that this may not provide the professional support required for the physiotherapist member of the team, and arrangements were made with the physiotherapy manager to retain regular contact and provide specific professional/peer support where necessary. Initially, the physiotherapist on the team did organise meetings with the physiotherapy department manager; however, over time, these reduced in frequency (at the individual's discretion) and she no longer meets with the manager. This may be due to a number of reasons: the team is very effective and works cohesively with each member acknowledging the value of others, regular reflection and informal supervision occurs, regular appraisal and development plans are agreed and there is regular contact with other physiotherapists on a day-to-day basis in the clinical areas. While maintaining their links with their previous peers, it is also very clear that each member of the team views themselves as an outreach practitioner, not as a critical care nurse or physiotherapist who works for an outreach service. The practitioners have created a very clear identity for themselves. This original concern regarding appropriate managerial and professional support has, therefore, not arisen.

Each practitioner brings their own individual strengths, although they all operate to the same job description and are able effectively to assess and manage an 'at risk patient'. As a whole, the team can deliver all of the skills that would be required for the range of level 0 to level 3 dependent patients (Intensive Care Society 2002) and continue to learn from and support each other.

Box 10.14 Lessons learned/tips for success

- Develop clear job descriptions and set role boundaries.
- Delegate clear levels of authority.

- Ensure that staff from multi-professional backgrounds are provided with appropriate professional support, e.g. negotiate time with other managers, encourage supervision sessions.
- Develop an environment of open discussion and debate.

AUDIT AND EVALUATION

Box 10.15

The main challenges identified include:

- auditing 'outreach' patients/services is highly complex;
- it is difficult to attribute improvements in care to one service;
- no nationally recommended dataset is available;
- effectively interpreting and managing the information obtained can be a challenge.

All clinicians are expected to participate in and, where appropriate, lead audit projects (DoH 1998). Monitoring and reviewing progress is a crucial means of checking whether plans are on target to achieve specific goals, and allows for revision and modifications where necessary (Wilson 1999; Banks 2002). While the audit data we have obtained is very encouraging, it is important to acknowledge the complex nature of auditing outreach services.

1. The outreach practitioner is not the only clinician involved in the care of the patient and, therefore, it is difficult to attribute any success to one individual service.
2. The thrust of outreach services is about preventing adverse events, so in effect, we are attempting to prove a negative (the adverse event did not happen because of our intervention, but how do we prove that it would have happened anyway?).
3. The impact of other developing services upon improvements in care, e.g. the development of a new six-bedded high-dependency unit will have impacted on patient care; however, it is difficult to separate out this effect from the outreach data.
4. Some situations are beyond the influence and control of the outreach team, e.g. bed management issues.
5. Anecdotally, the education provided to ward-based staff has resulted in improvements in care, however, this is extremely difficult to quantify.

A number of evaluative/audit approaches have therefore been used including:

- outreach team members' evaluations (including night nurse practitioners and the wider team);
- reflective practice;
- staff and patient satisfaction surveys;
- clinical audit database;
- incident monitoring;
- critical care staff feedback;
- senior clinicians' and managers' feedback.

Staff and patient satisfaction surveys have yielded encouraging information, some of which has been used to develop the service further. A patient satisfaction survey revealed that patients were not clear of our role or identity.

> 'I was visited at my bedside by various staff but cannot remember who they were.'
> ' I cannot remember who I was visited by . . .'

These comments were attributed, in part, to the team not having a uniform. A uniform is now worn by all staff on clinical duty providing a clear identity. The team also developed an information and advice leaflet that is given to patients and relatives following a prolonged stay in critical care.

In 2002, a questionnaire was sent to members of the multi-professional team who were viewed as colleagues and service 'users'. Staff were asked to identify the aspects of the service that were the most beneficial to them.

Physiotherapist:

- Very easy to contact and very approachable to ask for advice.
- Education, tracheostomy care and advice, fluid management.
- Safety mechanism: to assist in preventing patients' deterioration; often wards too busy to monitor poorly patients properly.

Senior house officer, surgery:

- To follow up patients post-ICU/HDU, discharge and advise on their management and assess patients who may need critical care involvement.

Staff grade:

- Link with ITU/HDU. Improved airway management.

Specialist registrar surgery:

• Have reduced rate of readmissions to ITU.

Staff nurse:

• Early response, appropriate help and practical assistance.

Some comments were made about the use of the early warning scoring system.

> Good in general but doesn't mean the same thing in every patient. Gives rise to unnecessary alarms. Some patients might trigger a high score while very simple measures would be enough to deal with underlying cause. (Specialist registrar)

Changes have been made to the system in accordance with staff comments and suggestions, resulting in a more user-friendly tool.

The team have developed their own audit database, which is used to evaluate the services provided against our key objectives, and to inform future developments. A recurring theme within the audit outcomes and recommendations is the need for more education and training.

In collaboration with the practice-based educator, formal and informal educational programmes are delivered and evaluated. A one-day 'Greater Manchester Acute Illness Management' course has been developed and is well attended and evaluated by all members of the multi-professional team.

The outreach practitioners are integral to the delivery of this and a number of other teaching sessions and study days.

Team members both deliver and receive education, dependent upon the subject matter. They also attend other educational events provided throughout the Trust, including sessions for medical, nursing and physiotherapy staff.

Box 10.16 Lessons learned and tips for success

• Plan what you will audit prior to the introduction of the service.
• Code all activities.
• Utilise any help available – administrative support, audit departments, junior staff projects.
• Promote and share audit results – good and bad.
• Close the loop – lack of feedback about implementation of recommendations is de-motivating.
• Acknowledge limitations and complexities.

The challenge for all critical care outreach services is to demonstrate the positive impact on patient outcomes. Due to the complex nature of 'at risk' and critically ill patients, accurate and meaningful data is difficult to obtain.

More detail regarding locally obtained audit data can be found in Chapter 13.

'POLITICAL' AWARENESS

Box 10.17

Main challenges include:

- political awareness raising among the team;
- understanding the concerns of others;
- developing effective strategies to deal with other professional colleagues.

There is a need for practitioners to be sensitive to the internal 'politics' within the hospital and the traditional hierarchical systems within which we work.

A small number of clinical staff felt somewhat threatened by the introduction of the outreach service; there was a perception that their clinical skills were being called into question, and they felt professionally undermined.

Individual professional groups may find the traditional hierarchies 'comfortable', and often perceive role development and new ways of working as a threat to their unique professional skills, knowledge and identity. Despite the modernisation agenda, there are very few examples of multi-professional team working and training. This unfamiliarity and lack of awareness of the benefits of a team approach can make clinicians wary and territorial (Herzberg 1999).

The introduction of the service heralded a challenge to the power status quo. Consultants traditionally retain overall responsibility for their patients and are the ultimate decision makers about their care. Understandably, they may have some concerns about the input of a new service into their patients' management. However, the system of care delivery in the new, modern health service can place unnecessary 'bottlenecks' in the patient's journey and result in delays in treatment (Cook et al. 2001). One of the key modernisation and outreach objectives is to instil a culture of professional and organisational cooperation and partnership working. This will improve communication, develop shared working practices and enhance patient care (Kenny 2002).

We regularly discuss our dealings with other professional groups, and make conscious decisions about the best way to handle certain situations in order to achieve our objectives. The team work collaboratively and exercise respectful assertiveness in order to overcome some of these problems.

Box 10.18

Lessons learned/tips for success.

• Don't assume everyone will think the same way as you do.
• Acknowledge and address the concerns of others.
• Try and look at things from the view point of others.
• Seize any opportunities to work collaboratively.
• Timing may be a key factor in the success or failure of new initiatives.

FUTURE CHALLENGES

A number of challenges need to be overcome in the future in order to ensure the ongoing successful development and integration of the critical care outreach services. Locally, these challenges include:

• 'flattening' the hierarchies and tackling professional elitism to ensure effective team and partnership working; modernising career pathways and multi-professional education and training will help to develop the right environment to ensure that multi-professional working in and across the team becomes the norm rather than the exception (DoH 2001; Glenn and Reeves 2004);
• the establishment of an evidence base (local and national) that supports the further development of critical care outreach;
• the development of a successful business case to ensure parity of service provision throughout the organisation.

From a national and strategic perspective, the future challenges that need to be addressed include:

• clarity around the delivery of critical care outreach services and parity in funding across the National Health Service;
• ensuring that legislation keeps pace with service development, e.g. the expansion of nurse and allied health professional prescribing;
• The impact of the European Working Time Directive and Modernising Medical Careers must be assessed in terms of provision of acute care over the twenty-four-hour time frame;
• workforce development plans and recruitment strategies should pay greater attention to the design, competencies and development of multi-professional teams that are enabled to speak a common language and develop patient driven solutions (DoH 2000f).

CONCLUSION

The provision of a seamless service demands collaboration and multi-professional working and learning (DoH 2000a). Modernisation of service delivery and provision has presented some exciting opportunities for new ways of working which, if managed effectively, can enhance the patient journey by pooling a diverse range of competencies to deliver a flexible and responsive service, focusing on patient need rather than particular professional aspects of care delivery.

Embracing the modernisation agenda in the delivery of services can present some unexpected challenges, not least of which is the difficulty in introducing change into a well-established system and organisational culture. The NHS has seen the introduction of numerous changes in the recent past, and each new idea seems to be met with a healthy degree of scepticism. Key to overcoming these genuine reservations of healthcare professionals is the careful, staged management of change – to keep it so subtle that the staff don't realise it is happening until it is achieved!

A major factor in ensuring the success of our service was the recruitment of the right team members – focusing on the skills, knowledge and attitude required by the team, rather than the individual team member and their professional identity.

Each profession has a unique contribution to make to the team effort. While acknowledging the overlap in the competencies of different healthcare professionals, other colleagues need to understand and accept the shift in emphasis from professional identities to a team focus. Each individual's different contributions must be valued and respected (DoH 2000f). Effective leadership and management arrangements should be directed towards maximising the impact and development of the concept of 'team' (DoH 2000a), celebrate our differences and seize any opportunities for shared learning and improvements in care.

REFERENCES

Banks C (2002) Make the most of your team. *Nursing Standard* 17(10): 96.
Belbin RM (1999) Management teams. *Why They Succeed or Fail*. Oxford: Butterworth-Heinemann.
Cook G, Gerrish K, Clarke C (2001) Decision making in teams: issues arising from two UK evaluations. *Journal of Inter Professional Care* 15(2): 141–51.
Cook I, Render M, Woods D (2000) Gaps in the continuity of care and progress on patient safety. *British Medical Journal* 320(7237): 791–5.
Department of Health (1998) *A First Class Service: Quality in the New NHS*. London: Department of Health.
Department of Health (1999) *Making a Difference: Strengthening the Nursing, Midwifery and Health Visiting Contribution to Health and Healthcare*. London: Department of Health.

Department of Health (2000a) *A Health Service of All the Talents: Developing the NHS Workforce*. London: Department of Health.
Department of Health (2000b) *Investment and Reform: Taking Forward the NHS Plan*. London: Department of Health.
Department of Health (2000c) *The NHS Plan: A Plan for Investment and Reform*. London: Department of Health.
Department of Health (2000d) *Comprehensive Critical Care. A Review of Adult Critical Care Services*. London: Department of Health.
Department of Health (2000f) *Working Together: Securing a Quality Workforce for the NHS*. London: Department of Health.
Department of Health (2000g) *Meeting the Challenge: A Strategy for the Allied Health Professions*. London: Department of Health.
Department of Health (2001) *Working Together, Learning Together*. London: Department of Health.
Freeman M, Miller C, Ross N (2000) The impact of individual philosophies of teamwork on multi professional practice and the implications for education. *Journal of Inter Professional Care* 14(3): 237–48.
Glenn S, Reeves S (2004) Developing inter professional education in the pre-registration curricula: mission impossible? *Nurse Education in Practice* 4: 45–52.
Herzberg J (1999) Tribes or teams? The challenge of multi professional education. *Hospital Medicine*. 60(7): 516–19.
Hill K, Ingala J (2001) Build a dream team. *Nursing Management* 22(9): 37–9.
Hyrkas K, Appelqvist-Schmidlechner K (2003) Team supervision in multi professional teams: team members' descriptions of the effects as highlighted by group interviews. *Journal of Clinical Nursing* 12: 188–97.
Intensive Care Society (2002) *Guidelines for the Introduction of Outreach Services*. ICS.
Kenny G (2002) Inter professional working: opportunities and challenges. *Nursing Standard* 17(6): 33–6.
McKinley S (2001) Critical care education is given a redesign. *Nursing Times* 97(27): 34–5.
Morey JC, Simon R, Gregory D, Wears RL, Salisbury M, Kimberley A et al. (2002) Error reduction and performance improvement in the emergency department through formal teamwork training: evaluation results of the med teams project. *Health Services Research* 37(6): 1553–81.
Outhwaite S (2003) The importance of leadership in the development of an integrated team. *Journal of Nursing Management* 11: 371–6.
Ovretveit J (1997) Leadership in multi professional teams. *Health and Social Care in the Community* 5(4): 269–83.
Reay T, Golden-Biddle K, Germann K (2003) Challenges and leadership strategies for managers of nurse practitioners. *Journal of Nursing Management* 11(6): 396–403.
Ridgway J, Maxwell E (2001) Clinical governance and you. *Nursing Times* 97(1): 36.
Risser D, Rice M, Salisbury M, Simon R, Jay G, Berns S (1999) The potential for improved teamwork to reduce medical errors in the emergency department. *Annals of Emergency Medicine* 34(3): 373–83.
Scholes J, Vaughan B (2002) Cross boundary working: implications for the multi-professional team. *Journal of Clinical Nursing* 11: 399–408.

Sheridan M (2003a) Clinical leadership: part 2. Transforming leadership. *Professional Nurse* 18(12): 716–17.

Sheridan M (2003b) Clinical leadership: part 3. How to foster a leading role for everyone. *Professional Nurse* 19(1): 56–7.

Simons F (2003) Clinical leadership: part 1. Key components of the programme. *Professional Nurse* 18(11): 656–7.

Spath P (2004) Taking charge when you're not in charge. *Hospital Case Management* 12(7): 111–12.

Truman P (2000) A question of style. *Nursing Management* 7(8): 10–12.

Vincent C, Neale G, Woloshynowych M (2001) Adverse events in British hospitals: preliminary retrospective record review. *British Medical Journal* 322(7285): 517–20.

Walton M (1984) Differing – to agree! *Nursing Mirror* 158(13): 26–7.

Williams J (2004) In the midst of difficulty lies opportunity. *Nursing Management* 11(4): 17–19.

Wilson J (1999) Clinical audit systems. *British Journal of Nursing* 8(12): 821–3.

10 Case study: the role of the physiotherapist in the critical care outreach team

ALEX LARKIN AND SALLY KNIGHTLY

INTRODUCTION

This chapter aims to describe the rationale behind the recruitment of a multi-professional team to provide a critical care outreach service within a district general hospital. Having been appointed to the role of the consultant nurse within critical care, and being allocated a budget to deliver outreach with respect to the 'comprehensive critical care philosophy', I was able to determine what competencies were required to meet both patient and service need (see Chapter 10 for more information). What follows is an honest account of thoughts and pre-conceived ideas of both myself, and the physiotherapist on the team (Sally Knightly). Prior to her appointment to the team both Sally and I had our own views about how we thought the role would be integrated and how it would develop over time. These views were always very fluid, and there was a 'suck it and see' approach, which has proven to be extremely useful in terms of developing the individual, the role, the team and the service.

Why did we seek to recruit a physiotherapist to the outreach team?

Consultant nurse's view

At the time of recruiting to our critical care outreach team, there had been a major investment in the 'comprehensive critical care' agenda, and numerous job opportunities were available, particularly for critical care nurses. We were attempting to recruit from a dwindling pool of highly skilled staff and therefore had to think creatively about who to target as suitable candidates. Having determined the competencies required of the critical care outreach practitioner, we realised that other healthcare professionals would be able to fulfil the role; in particular, we recognised that physiotherapists working within the

Critical Care Outreach. Edited by Lee Cutler and Wayne Robson.
Copyright 2006 by John Wiley & Sons Ltd.

field of critical care/respiratory medicine, would possess the range of skills and knowledge required for the post of critical care outreach practitioner. This belief was based on previous experiences of working with other professional groups, and having developed an understanding of their exceptional and often under-valued level of knowledge, skill and expertise. The posts were therefore advertised in nursing and physiotherapy journals in order to attract appropriate applicants.

A number of other factors also influenced my decision to recruit a physiotherapist. The political agenda of 'liberating the talents' and 'new ways of working' seemed to me to provide healthcare services with an ideal opportunity to work in a truly multi-professional manner. I felt that this would provide an exciting opportunity for cross-professional learning, and would stimulate and challenge nursing colleagues who have traditionally worked in professional silos. The addition of a physiotherapist, who would operate to the same job description as the nurses on the team, would, I hoped, serve to enhance the whole team competencies and ensure that there was a truly holistic approach to the spectrum of acute and rehabilitation care for our patients.

Another potential benefit would be that of developing or broadening career opportunities for senior physiotherapy staff. We have significant recruitment and retention issues for this particular staff group and, while it is acknowledged that we would potentially exacerbate this problem by recruiting to the team, I felt that, in the long run, the opportunity would be seen as a positive development and would provide another career pathway for those physiotherapists interested in acute care.

What factors influenced your decision to apply for the job?

Physiotherapist's view

I had been working with acutely unwell and critically ill patients within the critical care units and acute surgical wards for a number of years. I felt that the prospect of joining the outreach team would enable me to provide more holistic care and enable me to follow up the patient throughout the whole of their acute illness episode. I was aware of the developments and recommendations within 'comprehensive critical care' and felt that it presented the opportunity for multi-professional working within a team, rather than teams of individual professional groups working together.

Working within a multi-professional team would also help to break down professional barriers and allow me to further expand my role and develop my knowledge and skills, in particular, with respect to the follow-up care required for patients who have undergone critical care.

Having worked a traditional Monday–Friday 9–5 job, the prospect of working on a shift basis, which required cover from 7.45 am to 9 pm Monday to Sunday, was a new way of working for me, and I felt that it would fit well with the needs of my young family. This has proven to be a bonus of the role as I feel I would have struggled if I had continued to work my previous hours.

What were your expectations about having a physiotherapist in the team?

Consultant nurse's view

Including a team member from different professional background would hopefully fulfil my expectations on a number of levels. On a strategic level, I was keen to illustrate that the government agenda of working in new ways was achievable and could be integrated into the real world. While the strategic agenda emphasised the value of multi-professional teams, I was aware that, in the main, nurses had been appointed to outreach posts. While this seems appropriate, I felt that the outreach services risked losing the holistic approach required for the complex group of patients that we see. I was, therefore, very keen to see the whole team fulfilling the same job description of outreach practitioner, rather than having a physiotherapist 'on the team'.

Locally, this development has demonstrated to other physiotherapists that there are opportunities for role diversification, which is beneficial in terms of recruitment and retention. I also felt that there would be advantages to other team members (including myself) in terms of sharing skills, learning from each other, enhancing the whole team competencies and understanding the perspective of other professionals regarding what others see as a 'nursing' role. Effective integration of the team would hopefully break down professional barriers and improve communication with other staff within the clinical areas.

I anticipated some resistance to this initiative, particularly from nursing staff who may have felt that the posts should remain within nursing. This in fact did not occur, and Sally is accepted and respected by the clinical staff.

The personnel department had a number of issues with the job descriptions and advised that it would not be possible to use the same job description for the nursing staff as for the physiotherapist. After a number of conversations, this was resolved by developing two job descriptions – both identical in content except for the qualifications and details on the person specification!

On a practical level, I discussed issues with the management team around the potential barriers of traditional nursing skills being undertaken by a physiotherapist, for example drug administration, venepuncture, cannulation, managing central lines and providing advanced life support. These concerns were overcome by developing team policies and guidelines, influencing trust drug administration policies to include other staff groups, and attendance at appropriate training and education sessions (including the Resuscitation Council UK Advanced Life Support).

The reality of true multi-professional team working has surpassed my expectations. All team members have an excellent knowledge base, which they share willingly within and outside the team. There is an enhanced understanding of the work of other clinical teams, and frequent opportunities for learning new skills. Our working relationship with physiotherapists, speech and language therapists and dietitians is highly effective and has resulted in a number of initiatives to improve patient care.

What were your expectations about working on the team?

Physiotherapist's view

I have always worked within a multi-professional team and I enjoy sharing my knowledge and skills, while developing myself and learning new things. The development of the critical care outreach practitioner post was an exciting opportunity to use my skills and knowledge in a different way, taking on new responsibilities and developing the role of the physiotherapist in a new field.

What did other nurses think about the idea of a physio working in outreach?

Consultant nurse's view

The nurses within the team had no problems with the concept. The role and the service were new to all the team members and each individual required support. This support was two-way, not simply the nurses supporting the physiotherapist. In the early days, nursing staff outside the team seemed to have more difficulty in accepting the role. Junior nursing staff in particular seemed to show some resentment towards the role for reasons that are not entirely clear. Perhaps there were some professional issues around taking advice from a team member outside their professional group. It did appear that Sally had to 'prove' herself to the nursing staff, whereas the nurses on the team were accepted at face value. Perhaps this was due to their own lack of insight into the level of knowledge and skills of the physiotherapist. Sally has worked very hard to network and build up relationships with ward-based staff, and these issues now seem to have been resolved.

What did other physiotherapists think about the idea of a physiotherapist taking on the role of the outreach practitioner?

Physiotherapist's view

The general view of my colleagues was that this was an exciting opportunity that fully recognised the level of knowledge and skills possessed by a physiotherapist. While commenting that they were sorry to lose me, the managers were highly supportive of my application, and acknowledged that it may provide an alternative career pathway for acute physiotherapy staff.

How has your experience of working with the team compared with your expectations?

Joint view

We both feel, as do other members of the team, that the experience has been very positive. There has been much more sharing of skills and knowledge than either of us anticipated, resulting in a real passion for learning and development. The blurring of the professional boundaries had been achieved to such an extent that staff who do not know the individual team members are not aware of the professional backgrounds of each member. They all function at the same level and possess the same range of skills, though clearly each has their particular strengths and interests.

What advice would you give to other outreach teams who are considering employing physiotherapists or other allied health professionals?

Consultant nurse's view

Working in new ways has been a great success for us, and I am a strong advocate of this approach to healthcare delivery. While there may be some potential barriers, none of these is insurmountable and should not act as a deterrent.

One should consider the knowledge, skills and competencies that are required for the whole team and investigate who would possess these skills before deciding which professional group to recruit from. Traditional recruitment approaches persist in restricting professionals to a pre-defined role that potentially no longer meets service and patient needs. Simply adding a physiotherapist on to the team to undertake their traditional role was, in my view, a wasted opportunity to benefit the patient, the professions and the organisation. Using the same job title, i.e. critical care outreach practitioner, regardless of the professional background of the individual, has been very effective in clarifying the role for other members of staff.

The critical care outreach service is able to meet the needs of a range of complex patients. Where we do not possess the knowledge and skills ourselves, we will either aim to develop ourselves to meet these needs or refer appropriately to other professional groups. Working effectively within a team enables us to capitalise on our strengths and expose any weaknesses that need to be addressed. It is possible and indeed desirable to capitalise on opportunities for shared learning and development. This is achievable with the development of robust policies and governance arrangements which are designed to support and protect patients and individuals who are extending their scope of practice beyond the 'traditional' boundaries.

The introduction of new ways of working can throw up unexpected issues. Education may be required to influence the attitude of others who may be unaware of the benefits of this innovative approach. The individual may also require support until they feel established in the role, and part of my role is to act as a sponsor and advocate for the multi-professional team approach.

While the issue of peer support has not been a particular problem, it may be necessary to organise time out for peer supervision and/or attendance at meetings with staff from specific professional backgrounds in order to maintain professional links and keep updated with regard to profession specific issues.

What advice would you give to other physiotherapists or allied health professionals who are considering working within critical care outreach?

Physiotherapist's view

Working in new ways is an excellent development that provides many benefits. While acknowledging that there are a number of challenges in terms of introducing a new role, the opportunity to move and shape professional boundaries is highly rewarding. There is initially a temptation to stick within your 'comfort zone' and operate in the same 'physiotherapy' role. It is important to leave your previous role behind – delegate physiotherapy tasks where possible, but use the opportunity to teach and support junior colleagues.

One should be aware that it may not be plain sailing – there may be some issues that need to be addressed in order to ensure the success of the role. Do not work on the assumption that everyone else will think in the same way that you do. Promoting and selling the role to others may be necessary, in order to develop their understanding and acceptance.

I had some concerns initially regarding the loss of professional identity and the loss of clinical skills. To preserve my skills and keep contact with my 'roots', I have maintained a working relationship with my peer group, attend meetings locally and nationally and contribute to the delivery of training for junior colleagues. Being clinically based, I am also able to practise my professional skills, in the absence of a physiotherapist being available.

FINAL JOINT REFLECTIONS

Key to the success of the development of team competencies has been the shared learning that has occurred between the nursing and physiotherapy staff. These are highlighted in Table C10.1.

Initially, each team member approached the patient assessment in a slightly different way, with their focus being compatible with their individual area of

Table C10.1 Skills and knowledge the nurses and physiotherapist have developed and learned from each other

Learned by the physiotherapist	Learned by the nurses
• Pharmacology and drug administration	• Specialist clinical skills, e.g. humidification, patient positioning
• Cannulation	• Cannulation
• Priming an intravenous administration set	• Chest auscultation
• Advanced life support skills	• Advanced life support skills
• Interpretation of blood results	• Interpretation of blood results
• Rhythm recognition	• Neurological follow-up and rehabilitation
• Management of peripheral and central lines.	• Ordering chest X rays
• Ordering chest X rays	• Working under patient group directions
• Working under patient group directions	• Psychological care
• Psychological care	• Making appropriate referrals to physiotherapy
• Changing tracheostomy tubes	

expertise. Having worked together over the last three and a half years, the team have developed a standard approach to patient assessment and care delivery. Clinical decisions are based on patient need, and a holistic approach has been cultivated. Although not evidence-based, our perception is that no clear differences in patient assessment and management are apparent.

The traditional role of the physiotherapist requires them to have developed the ability to make clinical decisions when working alone. This was not the case for the nursing staff who were used to being able to discuss decisions and possible outcomes with other colleagues. The opportunity to do this may be limited as an outreach practitioner, and the support from the physiotherapist to develop this skill was invaluable.

Multi-professional team working has resulted in effective communication across all clinical teams, in particular, there is close liaison with physiotherapists, rehabilitation teams and access to follow-up services is enhanced.

A further development for the role of the physiotherapist has been the involvement in instigating and discussing do-not-attempt-resuscitation decisions. This was a new area for the physiotherapist and, while initially quite daunting, it has served to promote the delivery of holistic care.

CONCLUSION

Policy enablers have been used to maximum effect in order to deliver a successful multi-professional outreach service. Acknowledgement of strengths and weaknesses, shared learning and staff support has seen the development of a team that possesses a broad range and depth of clinical competencies. Creative recruitment strategies can deliver a number of benefits for the individuals involved, the patient and the organisation, and consideration should be given to this approach wherever possible.

11 The learning needs of critical care outreach practitioners

LEE CUTLER

INTRODUCTION

This chapter aims to consider the learning needs of critical care outreach practitioners across their career trajectory. Activities and strategies aimed at meeting these needs are also discussed. Examples and suggestions are shared in order that the chapter has practical applicability for the reader. The chapter refers to work undertaken by a network of outreach teams who have attempted to articulate and meet their own learning needs. Thus the chapter content is embedded in the reality of contemporary practice and, while some of the discussion relates to outreach generally, the chapter is to a great extent a case study in itself.

Those who work as outreach practitioners will find this chapter useful when considering their own development, as well as those they may be responsible for supervising and mentoring. Managers, educationalists and aspiring outreach practitioners may also find the chapter useful.

CURRENT CONTEXT

The learning needs and processes of critical care outreach practitioners have been given little consideration in the literature (Younker 2002) though the need to address these has been acknowledged (Coombs 2002). Where these needs are discussed in the literature there is some disagreement. Within the *National Outreach Report* (Modernisation Agency 2003) some suggestions for outreach skills were made, but it was acknowledged that local needs analysis is important. The report also acknowledged the great variation in models of practice nationally. The approach of matching knowledge and skills with models of practice, advocated in the report, seems appropriate given the national diversity in practice currently seen.

In contrast to this, others have advocated standardisation of aspects of outreach, not least the prerequisite education and ongoing development

Critical Care Outreach. Edited by Lee Cutler and Wayne Robson.
Copyright 2006 by John Wiley & Sons Ltd.

(Younker 2002). While there are many challenges in attempting standardisation and national competencies for critical care it seems increasingly likely that such standardisation will be a feature of critical care in the future (Scholes and Endacott 2003) and of advanced level practice throughout the registered paramedical health professions.

The current reality is that practitioners in the field need education, support and leadership in order to be successful and effective in this challenging area of practice. While there may be some disagreement about the ways this should be achieved there seem to be some broad principles and themes that are central when considering these issues.

Outreach was introduced to address a set of complex problems that exist within acute care areas. At the time of introduction the extent and nature of these problems was not fully appreciated and it is now evident that outreach is not a 'quick fix' but rather an element of a long-term solution (Coombs 2002). Practising on the current interface of acute and critical care and attempting to enhance the care of deteriorating or recovering critically ill individuals is one of the greatest challenges a critical care professional can face. The busy acute medical or surgical ward, for example, presents a stark contrast to the critical care unit. Critical care units comprise an expert community, high ratios of staff to patients and technological equipment ready to hand. Practising in the new sub-speciality of critical care outreach requires a range of knowledge and skills, personal qualities, professional maturity and 'hardiness' for practice as well as political and diplomatic savvy.

There was perhaps an assumption that being critical care trained would be 'enough' and that colleagues back in the ICU or HDU would always be there for support. Although critical care might be a sound foundation for outreach it has become clear that the range of skills and knowledge and the context in which they need to be applied differs substantially from the ICU or HDU. Working in a small team or alone in outreach may also set practitioners aside from the larger critical care community where the work is often more defined, more predictable, organised and observable.

Prior to the establishment of outreach services it was not possible to appreciate fully the support and development needs of staff working in these teams. But the lessons learned over the past few years should inform our future directions. Already nurses have left outreach and it is apparent that nurses who 'leave the comfort zone' of critical care require understanding, support and investment in their development.

While the current NHS human resource strategy aims to make explicit and support the development of key knowledge and skills for practice (DoH 1999) the NHS Knowledge and Skills Framework gives only a general guide.

As the KSF is a broad generic framework that focuses on the application of knowledge and skills – it does **not** describe the exact knowledge and skills that people need to develop. More specific standards/competences would help to do this as would the outcomes of learning programmes (DoH 2004, p. 6).

It is therefore imperative to articulate and share the specific knowledge and skills that are applied in this advanced role. It is also important to acknowledge not only the observable learning outcomes but also the value of engagement in a wide range of learning processes (Milligan 1998) and the more tacit benefits that come from sharing experiences and discussing the complexities and dilemmas of daily practice (Fulbrook 2004). The latter is especially important since problems seen in practice do not always present themselves as well formed structures – rather they are often messy, indeterminate situations (Schon 1987). These require critical thinking, inventiveness and improvisation.

The remainder of this chapter will consider some of the key stages in the career path of critical care outreach practitioners. In doing this a perspective on the knowledge and skill needed in outreach will be presented. There will also be some consideration of the indeterminate, complex and contentious nature of practice in outreach that has emerged through discourse between practitioners working in outreach.

CAREER DEVELOPMENT IN CRITICAL CARE OUTREACH

Moves to formalise career pathways for healthcare professionals in the National Health Service have been in evidence in recent years. The Department of Health has called for career pathways to be made explicit within critical care nursing (DoH 2001). One could argue that Agenda for Change (DoH 1999) and the NHS Knowledge and Skills Framework (DoH 2004) have added greater substance and structure to the career trajectories of nurses and allied health professionals in critical care.

Critical care outreach has emerged as a further limb of the critical care career pathway. However, at present outreach is immature and more time and work is needed to consolidate current initiatives and experiences. Because of the limitations that are a feature of this immaturity, the remainder of this chapter concentrates on a simplistic view of the key stages in the outreach career trajectory with the aim of considering the learning challenges practitioners face at different stages (see Figure 11.1). It is not the intent here to prescribe or accurately represent the current reality; rather it is to indicate some of the key challenges and to give some structure to the discussion that follows. It is hoped that it may generate some reflection, critical thought and debate among readers.

While it is acknowledged that several professional groups are involved in outreach the discussion here focuses on non-medical practitioners

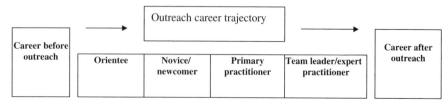

Figure 11.1 Key stages in the outreach career trajectory.

though this section may be of interest to all groups of staff involved in outreach.

CAREER BEFORE OUTREACH

Many will share an interest in, and hold opinions on, the essential prerequisites for outreach practice. The diversity in practitioners, job descriptions and clinical/Agenda for Change grades does not merely represent the different funding secured by individual critical care departments. It indicates that different ideologies and values also play a part.

Arguably, articulating the range of personal qualities, knowledge and skills required for outreach practice would help with better preparation for practice in the future. Such preparation helps career progression and makes sense in human resource terms. There are, however, many complex issues concerning how best to prepare professionals for practice. This has resulted in very significant changes in the types of curricula and programmes of education recently seen in the disciplines of nursing and medicine, for example. At the risk of being overly simplistic one could argue that in the case of areas such as critical care outreach one cannot completely pre-prepare for such a role since much essential learning has to take place in practice. However, examples of preparation for practice in outreach have been discussed in the literature and often focus on clinical skills and knowledge (see for example Anderson et al. 2002).

When outreach was emerging it was perhaps assumed that training and experience within critical care units are essential prerequisites for outreach practice. Critical care experience often allows the development of skills and knowledge that should be at the centre of clinical practice in outreach. However, there are drawbacks too. There are cases where acute ward nurses have been appointed as outreach practitioners. One such nurse related that:

> I approach situations in a different way ... I have an understanding of what is realistic in the context of a busy ward. (Anonymous outreach nurse)

The steepest learning curve for ICU nurses who venture on to the ward is around what is achievable in the context of a shortage of nursing staff, medical staff, equipment and critical care knowledge and skills among ward staff. However, the nurse also admitted that she lacked knowledge and skills that a critical care background would have given her. Clearly a team should have a range of practitioners who make unique and individual contributions. There is room in any team for individual strengths and weaknesses – what matters is that common values in the team mean that they share their expertise and perspective with others who lack it.

In Alex Larkin's chapter on the challenges of managing outreach she shares her perspective on the essential knowledge, attitude and skills she looked for in potential team members. These may guide those who have an interest in becoming an outreach practitioner and those who are looking to appoint team members. While many nurses were initially keen to work in outreach it is possible that the future expansion of outreach and critical care in general puts pressure on the human resource 'market' such that further recruitment to the role will be made difficult. In future, recruiting outreach practitioners from a range of clinical and professional backgrounds will strengthen and enrich critical care nationally. Alex Larkin's case study of employing a physiotherapist within the team serves as an example that could be considered by other teams. Box 11.1 below gives some suggestions for ensuring outreach will be accessible to multi-disciplinary practitioners in the future.

Box 11.1 Strategies for improving future recruitment to outreach

- Making explicit what knowledge and skills are required for undertaking the role.
- Formalising and making explicit what can be learned through outreach placements/shadowing and the ways in which students will learn while with outreach.
- Ensuring that outreach is part of acute and critical care placements for pre-registration staff.
- Ensuring that outreach is part of the training for post registration acute and critical care staff.
- Offering an outreach rotation/secondment as a development opportunity with the career development pathway for acute and critical care staff.
- Having a multi-disciplinary team approach to outreach that invites and values the different professional practitioners who can be part of an outreach team.
- Having person specifications that focus on evidence of competence rather than assuming competence through specific experience or professional background.

Preparatory learning for outreach practice should focus on the competencies that are core to the role of caring for critically ill patients and their families, as well as a depth and breadth of professional knowledge and higher academic and critical thinking abilities. One would hope that innovators continue to develop and share programmes and methods of learning and refine and expand the elementary work already undertaken.

INDUCTION AND ORIENTATION TO OUTREACH

Prior to consideration of the development needs within the role it is important to give some thought to the process of induction and orientation of the newly appointed outreach nurse. For many of those who pioneered outreach there was limited opportunity for this. but there is no excuse for a poor induction of a newcomer to an established team.

Introducing people to their new areas of work is extremely important. The risk is that once people have been appointed, the keenness of the appointing organisation to impress subsides and the agenda switches to ensuring that the new appointee is 'up and running' as soon as possible. Ensuring that people know how they will be supported is extremely important. Making a good start in this area means ensuring there is a comprehensive induction for new staff. Box 11.2 summarises the essentials of a good induction.

Box 11.2 Essentials of a good induction

- You have protected time to learn the basics and orientate yourself.
- You have a structured programme/list of things to familiarise yourself with.
- You are given the resources you need to fulfil the requirements of the role and are helped to become familiar with them.
- You have a named mentor/supervisor/resource person and are allocated time to spend with them.
- The people orientating you reflect on what it was like to be new and make every reasonable effort to help.

There should be systems in place to ensure that new appointees have a formal structured induction and orientation. This will ensure that the practitioner is helped to settle in and begin practising as soon as possible. Feeling new and disorientated is inevitable but familiarising the newcomer with local practices, policies and resources can help this. The list below contains key points drawn from the induction programme in my own Trust. It is used to structure the activity of the newcomer and those who act as their mentor. Some orientees prefer to find things out for themselves and be simply guided by the list. Others like written information to be provided or a discussion where information is shared verbally. Our team at Doncaster includes a training post for a Foundation SHO and since there is a new one joining the team every three or four months the following list has proved to be very helpful:

- team members and team structure
- awareness of shift times, patterns and formulation of duty rotas, sickness and annual leave policies
- who you are professionally and managerially accountable to
- organisational structure – departments, directorates
- system of appraisal, mentorship and clinical supervision
- service coverage (which clinical areas)
- methods of communicating (within the team, within the department/directorate/division, within the Trust, outside the Trust)
- location and contacts for key areas (wards, departments, specialist professionals)
- use of information technology (e-mail account, internet access, intranet access)
- hospital systems (e.g. pathology results, PAS)
- role and role boundaries
- protocols, policies and practice guidelines
- track and trigger system in use
- education provided by the team (formally and informally) and your role in its delivery
- equipment used by the team and use taught by team (transfer equipment, portable monitors, manometers)
- audit and service evaluation
- receiving referrals
- undertaking follow-up
- awareness of emergency procedures (cardiac arrest, how and where else to get help in other urgent situations)
- mandatory education (fire, cardiac arrest, moving and handling patients).

MAINTAINING CRITICAL CARE TEAM MEMBERSHIP

It is surprising to see how quickly colleagues are viewed as being outside the team once they are no longer on the ICU duty rota. Perceptions and beliefs about them change as do beliefs about the importance and validity of their work. Therefore maintenance of links with and membership of ICU/HDU community is a valid concern. This may be the source of some anxiety and planning how to address this issue during induction may be appropriate. There may be some formal arrangement for this such as critical care meetings that incorporate outreach. But nurses can be a cliquey bunch and maintaining good inter-team working relationships requires willingness on both sides.

There is value in allowing critical care nurses from ICU and HDU to spend some time with the outreach team. Only through experience can one begin to appreciate the demands and stresses of the role and the way different knowledge and skills are needed. Most important is an appreciation of how the different sub-groups of critical care can support each other.

Outreach practitioners may also feel it is important to maintain, or develop, ICU skills and knowledge. Methods for maintaining critical care links and knowledge and skills through clinical experience vary from one hospital to another; below is a list of just a few that have been employed:

• posts that involve rotation between outreach and ICU/HDU;
• annual update periods (e.g. two weeks on ICU);
• flexible arrangement so that when outreach workload allows, time is spent on ICU 'floating', helping out and teaching/supervising junior staff.

The best model is one that meets individual and local service needs. The models presented here have delivered some success but have also changed over time.

KNOWLEDGE AND SKILLS FOR THE ROLE

It is not the aim of this section to offer a comprehensive consideration of the progression from novice to expert in outreach. However, this spectrum of practice and professional development is acknowledged as being a likely reality within contemporary practice. Rather the major aim of this section is to consider broadly the learning needs of those who are working within outreach. This will be done through the presentation and discussion of a set of competencies. The competencies are indicative rather than comprehensive and reflect the concerns and focus of a group of outreach nurses with experience in the role (Box 11.3). The framework has limitations and is presented here as a preliminary piece of work for interest rather than as a prescription for practice. Furthermore attempting to validate these highlighted some disagreement and raised some interesting and contentious issues. These are discussed in brief below.

Box 11.3 How were the competencies developed?

• Outreach nurses in the North Trent Critical Care Network had been meeting regularly as a group since the establishment of their roles within seven hospitals in the area.
• Support and development had been highlighted as key reasons to carry on meeting in the long term. It was perceived that these needs would be best met in a structured way and so an event to identify learning needs was planned.

- A focus group was conducted and 22 nurses who worked in outreach attended. The nurses had between two months and three years' experience in outreach. They were all F or G grade with the exception of two who were consultant nurses.
- The nurses were each asked to reflect on their experiences in outreach and from this to identify areas of competence that they thought were important to their role. They were also asked to present examples to explain how these were relevant and important to the role. Each proposal was then discussed within the group and consensus reached as to whether it was valid within outreach practice and in what way the knowledge and/or skill proposed would be applied within the role.
- The areas identified by the group were used to formulate statements of learning outcome. These were intended to reflect the learning that would have taken place if the statement had been achieved. They were also written in a way that describes practice rather than abstract ways of knowing and thus the learning was focused on clinical competence. The statements were organised into key domains according to their focus:

    - patient focus
    - communication and interpersonal
    - healthcare systems and principles
    - service development, support and evaluation
    - professional learning

- An attempt was then made to validate these by anonymous postal questionnaire distributed to all those who attended the focus group; 50% of the nurses returned completed questionnaires indicating whether they agreed with the statements. A 'comments' box also allowed for opinions to be elaborated and explained.
- There was agreement with almost all the statements; however, some of the statements were contentious. Areas where there was disagreement are discussed below within the individual domains.
- The general theme from the additional comments recorded on the validation questionnaire was an acknowledgement that to possess all these would not be the norm but it would be something that the individuals could work towards and could use to structure and guide their development. It was also stressed that these competencies were additional to those that might be associated with significant experience and/or training in ICU practice for example.

The importance and relevance of each of the domains of competence are explained here. Suggestions are also made for how practitioners may develop within each domain. It is not the intention to suggest that there are specific ways of learning in the areas presented. This would be overly simplistic, since learning is a complex business. No one who understands this complexity would ever suggest that if you do X you will learn Y. However, some suggestions have been made. These suggestions are based on the shared experiences of numerous outreach and critical care practitioners and it is hoped they will stimulate the reader to debate, think critically and experiment with different approaches to and methods of learning.

PATIENT FOCUS DOMAIN

Box 11.4 Competencies

In promoting and role modelling best practice in the identification and care of critically ill patients and their families, the practitioner:

1. employs a systematic approach to situations involving seriously ill patients;
2. responds in a timely and effective manner to alterations in a patient's condition correctly employing urgent or emergency interventions when necessary;
3. applies a systematic and effective approach to health interviews and history taking;
4. utilises inspection, auscultation, percussion and palpation appropriately during clinical examination of patients;
5. appropriately requests or advocates, and accurately interprets, a range of relevant diagnostic tests and investigations;
6. applies advanced clinical skills and role expansion appropriate to patient needs and the clinical situation;
7. makes appropriate clinical judgements and decision making in relation to the clinical condition of patients and the need for therapeutic intervention;
8. according to medical prescription and/or within own scope of practice initiates, manages and evaluates a range of therapeutic interventions including medical technology and pharmacological therapies, demonstrating a comprehensive knowledge of their mechanism and safe use;
9. clearly communicates and documents clinical findings and advocated plans for action;
10. through critical awareness of emotional and psychological disorders and reactions in the critically ill and their families advocates/demonstrates appropriate management and/or referral to specialist professionals.

Critical care outreach practitioners spend a significant part of their time in clinical practice. Therefore, competencies in this domain are of critical importance if patients are to be resuscitated, prevented from deteriorating and helped in their recovery. The competencies are reflective of the advanced knowledge and skills that are required for this demanding role. They enable the outreach practitioner to intervene, and teach by demonstration and role modelling, through which there will be enhanced credibility.

When the nurses discussed and commented on this domain, and the competencies, there were several key issues of contention. First, some practitioners argued that they tried at all costs not to intervene because they espoused a model of outreach that was primarily advisory and educative, rather than 'interventionist'. However, they admitted that, at times, it was practically impossible and unethical not to intervene in some way. There is clearly a conflict here between the espoused model of practice and that which clinical situations demand, especially those that are urgent or an emergency. In discussing the reality of outreach practice Anderson et al. (2002) acknowledge that: 'Our expectations of being supportive, educational and advisory proved to be both naïve and idealistic.' It could be argued that it is imperative for the educator/advisor to be clinically credible and competent. It is important not least because a very powerful way of teaching about the assessment and management of critical illness is to role model and demonstrate (Davies 1993; Charters 2000).

A further issue, for the nurses who shared their views, was with regard to competency 4. The terminology used was culturally unfamiliar to some, though the ones who questioned the competency statement admitted that they did 'look', 'listen' and 'feel' in their assessments of patients. When the same nurses were asked to prioritise what an educational programme for outreach nurses should include, physical assessment skills were seen as a priority. There is an evident paradox here. Perhaps also reflected is an insecurity or lack of confidence in physical assessment skills rather than denial of their importance. It has been acknowledged that, for nurses, while physical assessment has been limited historically within the United Kingdom context, it is a developing domain of practice and can have positive effects on patient care within outreach practice (Coombs and Moorse 2002).

Because of the issues mentioned above concerning the espoused model of practice, the nurses were also divided on the issue of how they should expand their role. Among the group some nurses had done far less in terms of expanded roles since they had left the critical care unit. However, others had expanded their role further in performing roles such as intravenous cannulation, arterial puncture for blood sampling, administration and titration of oxygen and intravenous fluid by patient group direction. The perceived local needs of the service and the patients seemed to have been a major factor determining role expansion; however, it is clear that the espoused model of practice is also key.

Competence statements such as those above can be used to generate evidence in portfolio assessed courses, for example, or as part of the appraisal process for the NHS KSF, which will require demonstration of knowledge and skills used in practice. Figure 11.2 shows an example of a learning contract currently in use. It was developed to guide practice and assessment of competence in an area that may cause some anxiety for those who do not have extensive experience. A call from concerned ward staff could make a wide range of demands on the outreach practitioner.

The learning contract was developed through a mapping exercise. It highlights the standards of practice that should be aimed for and can guide the learner in this activity. It allows the provision of structured feedback to members of the team who have been orientated but who are developing within this domain. The form shows how, in reality, the patient focus domain competencies are integrated with other domains such as communication and professional learning.

A highly effective way of learning while working in practice is through work-based learning (Flannagan et al. 2000). Having a clinical mentor and engaging in supervised clinical practice that focuses on each element of the domain competencies allows for demonstration and practice of skills and decision-making with immediate feedback.

COMMUNICATION AND INTERPERSONAL DOMAIN

Box 11.5 Competencies

In facilitating a collaborative approach to care, the practitioner:

1. employs a range of effective communication strategies and interpersonal skills when interacting with patients, their family and other multi-disciplinary professionals;
2. utilises effective and appropriate leadership and follower skills in a range of clinical and non-clinical situations;
3. recognises and utilises effective and appropriate persuasion and influencing skills in a range of clinical and non-clinical situations;
4. provides balanced and supportive feedback to fellow practitioners and other healthcare professionals;
5. contributes to the work of a range of groups within health care demonstrating effective facilitation of meetings and skills of debate.

Learning Contract
'Clinical Consultation and Patient Review'

Practitioner: _____

Assessor: _____   Date of assessment: ___/ ___/ ___

Behavioural elements of competence	Evidence	Assessor
1. Receives referral/consultation, eliciting necessary information from the referring individual.[1,2]		
2. Responds in a timely, professional and appropriate manner whilst considering other demands and priorities.[1,2] (Attendance and/or telephone advice)		
3. On arrival in the referring clinical area – introduces self to staff and makes clear the purpose of the visit.[1]		
4. Gathers preliminary information to aid with review of patient and assessment of the need for immediate intervention.[1,2]		
5. Introduces self to patient (and family if present) and makes clear the purpose of the visit.[1]		
6. Systematically assesses the patient: • Physical examination[1,2] • History & health interview[1,2] • Notes & charts[1,2] • Investigations & results[1,2]		
7. Makes appropriate clinical judgements regarding the patient's condition, need for further investigations, further interventions, referrals & future review.[1,2]		
8. Intervenes/arranges/advises on appropriate intervention where necessary.[1,2]		
9. Requests appropriate investigations, or advises other practitioners to arrange these when outside own scope of practice.[1,2]		
10. Communicates effectively with the patient (& family) throughout.[1]		
11. Communicates effectively with the nursing staff in the ward/unit throughout.[1]		
12. Communicates effectively with Medical staff and AHPs throughout.[1]		
13. Appropriately documents findings, advice, referrals, events, untoward incidents etc.[1]		
14. Identifies knowledge/skill deficit in others and self and takes full advantage of opportunities for teaching/ learning.[1,2]		
Additional Comments:		

Mandatory Evidence for competency elements [1] - Direct observation
Mandatory Evidence for competency elements [2] - Question & Answer/explanation

Figure 11.2 Learning contract outlining the competencies relevant for clinical consultation and patient review in outreach. (Reproduced with permission of Critical Care Outreach Team – Doncaster and Bassetlaw Hospitals NHS Foundation Trust.)

Outreach practitioners work with a wide range of professionals. They also care for patients with diverse communication needs and challenges. Therefore they need to be great communicators, persuaders, decision brokers and diplomats. There is a need for all situations to be 'win–win', and in organisations where power within and between professions remains pervasive this is a great challenge. Furthermore, outreach is teamwork – but the teams with which, and within which, practitioners work are numerous and complex. Practitioners often need to switch between the roles of leader and follower dynamically and appropriately.

Without these skills and qualities there is great scope for communication failure within practice. The results include misunderstanding, conflict, fragmentation of care, and intervention and decision-making not based on accurate information. The results of these undoubtedly affect the patient as well as working relationships among professionals.

In discussing this domain practitioners unanimously affirmed their belief in the importance of these competencies to the role. This reflects the way in which effective outreach services are reliant upon the interpersonal skills of the team members. These competencies are supportive and facilitative of those in the patient focus domain. However, development within this domain offers a different challenge since it is linked with our own personal qualities, confidence, habits, behaviour and relationships – things that are built and shaped over time.

Perhaps the starting point for development in this domain is to find a trusted and expert mentor and negotiate appraisal and coaching of personal leadership, communication and interpersonal skills. Another way is to use peer observation and critique. This is often used among teachers and I have experimented with this in my own development in the clinical, leadership and teaching elements of my role. The approach used is outlined in a guidance sheet adapted from Brookfield (1995) and presented in Box 11.6.

Box 11.6 Peer observation and critique: explanatory notes

Why? – It may at first seem threatening to ask another to critique an aspect of your practice however, as Brookfield (1995, p. 83) notes 'colleagues' observations of our practice can be one of the most helpful sources of critical insight to which we have access'.

How? – Arrange for you and a peer to work together or for them to shadow and observe you. Tell people around you about the session. If this means attending meetings together, for example, ensure all present understand the reason for the reviewer's presence. If this involves being in on a teaching session ensure that those in the audience know.

Some points to make the process less painful:

1. Seek out a colleague who has significant experience in the area where you work/want to improve.
2. Don't take on too much or try to fit too much into a session. Quality will generate more detailed and constructive feedback than if you pack too much into the day/session.
3. Seek out someone who can communicate clearly.
4. Seek out someone who has a history of supporting colleagues struggling to improve their practice. (*This may be an informal role they perform or a skill they have – it doesn't have to be a teacher or formal mentor or supervisor.*)
5. Give clear instructions to your colleague regarding what you want them to look for. It could be that you want them to give their general impression of your approach. Or you may wish them to focus on something specific.
6. Try to make this process reciprocal – this means you observing/critiquing them at a later date. Not only will this help you think about attributes and abilities, but will also avoid any undesirable power dynamics and the presumption that one has a monopoly on wisdom.

Examples of problems you may perceive that could be used to direct the observation:

- An area of your work that you are experiencing problems with.
- An area where you have little experience.
- Feedback from a leadership/management/teaching programme highlighting areas in which you need to improve.

Giving feedback to others*:*

In order that the feedback is helpful and not destructive try to do the following things:

1. Be balanced; point out what went well before pointing out what needs further work.
2. Frame critical comments in terms of your own experience/difficulties/problems.
3. Be concrete when commenting on actions – use examples observed.
4. Suggest future activities or follow-up so that this is not just a one-off session.
5. Suggest others who you think may be able to help or give another perspective.

HEALTHCARE SYSTEMS AND PRINCIPLES DOMAIN

Box 11.7 Competencies

In practising effectively within complex systems and organisations, the practitioner:

1. differentiates and evaluates 'interventionist' and 'educative/supportive' models of outreach practice and utilises an appropriate balance of these in a range of clinical situations;
2. recognises models and systems of consultation and referral, and utilises local systems to ensure effective team working and appropriate intervention according to clinical need;
3. utilises organisational resources, as well as professional and clinical networks in the support and development of the service;
4. interprets legal, professional and ethical frameworks using these as a guide for practice as well as describing practices that fall outside the principles of these frameworks.

Like many other health professionals, Outreach practitioners operate within complex organisational and professional systems. Some of the systems within which they work are formal with explicit rules of conduct while others are informal with more tacit or variable determinants of acceptable behaviour and practice. Such systems present dilemmas for practitioners because of their inherent complexity, inconsistency, conflict and contradiction. By its very nature outreach raises dilemmas since its core concern is to address the results and causes of failures in the system.

One example of this is the difference between medical and surgical wards and clinical teams. I can support this claim with nothing more than anecdotal evidence, but at the risk of stereotyping would argue that the reality facing outreach practitioners is one where physicians and surgeons have different historical relationship with critical care generally and this affects collaboration with outreach.

It is essential that the practitioner can think critically about these models and systems in operation in health care and the concepts and principles on which they are based. This amounts to a cultural, professional, ethical and political awareness.

These abilities are the prerequisite for practice that is contextually appropriate. In this domain the guiding principles of critical care outreach are acknowledged. It is a feature of contemporary teams that they range from those who are purposely interventionist to those who avoid intervention and who are purposely educative and advisory in their operation. However, I would argue that to operate exclusively in either mode is to neglect the benefit of the other. The expertise in practice is about recognising when either mode should determine practice and also when they should be used together as they can be mutually facilitative.

It was clear from the discussion around this domain that it is difficult always to have clarity on guiding principles that should be used in individual situations as there is often conflict between teams, agendas and priorities. Furthermore, seeing where one fits within the system and or how best to 'position' oneself on key issues often requires expert judgement. In this sense outreach is highly 'political' and so outreach practitioners need an understanding of and good judgement about the 'politics' of health care local to them. However they also need to understand what principles apply regardless of politics, cultures, etiquette and systems. Thus they need to interpret ethical, professional and legal principles and how they are universally applicable.

Some teams, or individuals, may be more political or contentious than others. And learning within this domain should be locally and individually determined. This is a challenging area of learning and outside of academic courses work-based methods are valuable in the development of insight and awareness. Individual judgement and action require coaching which should include at least praise and constructive feedback, and to this end good mentorship is invaluable. Lastly critical reflection on our 'mistakes' is also very valuable, while criticism is not and neither is self-deprecation or blame. Everyone makes mistakes and working in the politically charged NHS means that power is rife and everyone will be offended or upset at some point.

SERVICE DEVELOPMENT, SUPPORT AND EVALUATION DOMAIN

Box 11.8 Competencies

In facilitating the development and delivery of an effective service, the practitioner:

1. effectively plans and manages change to improve service delivery and clinical care;
2. utilises a systematic approach to audit and service evaluation, appropriately interpreting data and producing clear concise reports/presentations for relevant audiences;
3. appraises models and systems for standard setting and benchmarking, and employs these appropriately in practice;

---

4. reviews current evidence relating to a range of clinical issues and makes appropriate recommendations for practice;
5. utilises a range of information technology in executing all elements of the role;
6. effectively manages human resources and sets priorities for activity.

Outreach evolved in the context of the modernisation agenda within the NHS. Service development and evaluation are increasingly more 'culturally normal'. The numerous published papers about outreach implementation, development and evaluation in the NHS and the emergence of the 'sharing event' also testify to the growing culture of innovation and willingness to share best practice in outreach.

The novelty of outreach has meant that, to meet the needs of patients in this dynamic area of practice, services have had to develop significantly since their inception. Those who have been involved with setting up outreach services will testify that there are definite phases in this process each shaped by different priorities and goals.

Because of its nature and focus outreach highlights and challenges inefficiencies in systems and practice. However, it is often difficult, in the context of busy acute and critical care services, to find the time to address these issues. There is a critical issue here of balance between intervention 'on demand' and the support, education and empowerment of clinical areas. Responding to urgent and important calls for help is not in question. However, the principle remains that outreach aims to prevent deterioration and it is a commonly held belief that the right activity, targeted appropriately at clinical areas and staff, helps to prevent system failures. But this demands time allocation within daily or weekly schedules for evaluation, planning, preparation and relationship building. Without this services face the prospect of merely 'firefighting'.

In discussing this domain practitioners were in unanimous agreement about its importance and the competencies were seen as a prerequisite for success. Practitioners who are unable to evaluate and develop services, or change their practice following interpretation of contemporary evidence, risk failure in this domain, the result of which is stasis and an inability to respond to the changing context and demands of critical care.

The ability to interpret a complex array of evidence, especially as it is presented in the literature, is facilitated by academic courses with a research focus. However, learning in this domain is also about learning from practice by reviewing evidence from practice, including the experiences of staff and patients as well as more measurable variables and outcomes. Work-based learning, through service improvement projects, facilitated and mentored by those with expertise in this field, is extremely valuable. In this way experience is shared and vicarious lessons may be learned without some of the frustration that can be associated with attempting to change practice.

Chapter 13 provides some points on audit in critical care outreach. Also there is a case study following Chapter 2 that shows how one outreach team have used audit to improve recognition of seriously ill patients. The beginning point for these improvements has correctly been to seek a thorough understanding before making any changes to the service or their practice. This avoids identifying the solution before an understanding of the problem has been achieved.

PROFESSIONAL LEARNING DOMAIN

Box 11.9 Competencies

In effectively facilitating learning, the practitioner:

1. analyses clinical strengths and weaknesses of other healthcare professionals, providing affirmation or intervening to support, as appropriate;
2. plans learning activities according to the needs of the learners;
3. utilises a variety of strategies to facilitate and evaluate learning in a range of healthcare professionals in diverse situations;
4. analyses own strengths and weaknesses and strives to address own weakness, as well as sharing strengths with others;
5. demonstrates the ability to learn from clinical experience and reflection as well as articulating the learning to others and relating its relevance to professional practice;
6. utilises a range of strategies and resources to maintain up-to-date and evidence-based practice;
7. demonstrates a proactive approach to career planning and the development of a balanced and appropriate professional portfolio.

The domain of professional learning is important for outreach staff as well as for the staff that outreach practitioners aim to support. The competencies within this domain, which are about helping others learn, will often constitute a significant amount of time within the role. This may be through engagement in planned activity as well as making the most of ad hoc opportunities to learn as they arise.

The reality is that better education is not the definitive solution to the problems seen in caring for seriously ill patients in the acute care environment. Human and technological resource shortages as well as the need for cultural and organisational change are also at the heart of the difficulties currently seen. However, education is part of the solution and outreach practitioners are faced with the challenge of helping acute care staff develop their critical care knowledge and skills. This will be a long-term endeavour and with it goes the challenges faced by all teachers who attempt to facilitate learning among practitioners in any practice-based discipline.

Regardless of how technically competent individual teachers are and how well-planned learning activities are, to learn individuals need ongoing support in practice. This support is often difficult to find because of the time and resource constraints on the ward. Secondly the ongoing follow-up support for learning at bedside is not given the status it deserves in cultures where there is an assumption that teaching means 'telling' and where telling results in learning. Learning is a process not an outcome. The real challenge, therefore, is how to develop a culture and environment that supports learning. An answer to this question is far beyond the scope of this discussion, nevertheless it important to acknowledge here that collaboration, a strategic approach, and adequate resources are essential within the hospital setting.

Discussions with outreach practitioners in the field have revealed several dilemmas which may have wider resonance. When aiming to help practitioners learn about something which will be applied in their clinical role there is a dilemma. It is about whether the teaching and learning should take place away from practice or whether it should take place in and through practice. One might argue that some of each is ideally required. But the real challenge is to achieve the right balance. A further concern is with the extent to which one should teach general principles or 'rules' when contextual factors and the need for individual judgements and solutions are evidently necessary in the complexity of clinical practice.

The realisation of these challenges is even more stark when the teacher is a practitioner. This is because it is difficult to take to the 'hard high ground' (Schon 1987) full of idealism and principle when one has to face the demands and complexities of acute care in contemporary health care.

Becoming an effective teacher requires confidence and an ability to plan teaching activity according to the needs of the learner, the topic or skill being taught, as well as the facilities and resources available. This only comes with extensive experience. But three key activities that can help in developing as a teacher are presented in Box 11.10.

Box 11.10 Activities to help in becoming a better teacher

Receiving coaching with key elements of teaching: Experienced teachers can offer very useful tips and suggestions about successful teaching. For example, one of the commonest reasons why novice teachers have negative classroom or clinical experiences is because of inadequate planning. Developing one's ability to lesson plan is invaluable in setting learning outcomes, selecting appropriate methods and breaking down the subject, the session and the group into manageable parts.

Peer and mentor observation: This involves being observed while teaching. This is extremely useful if constructive feedback is given and acted upon. It provides us with an insight into things that we may not notice or it may provide alternative views to those which our bias and inexperience maintains. A valuable complement to being observed is observing an experienced teacher and critically reflecting upon aspects of their teaching.

Keeping a log of teaching and periodically reviewing it: This involves attempting to build up a range of teaching experience using different approaches, teaching different sizes of group, different mixes of learners and teaching different topics and skills.

Reflections and shared experiences appear to challenge the assumption that having intensive care experience and/or training is adequate preparation for outreach practice. Regardless of previous experience and training entering outreach as a newcomer augurs a steep learning curve.

This chapter goes only part of the way towards acknowledging the nature and extent of knowledge and skill required to fulfil the demands of the role. But from the areas of competence identified in this section it is clear that there are major areas where the nurses involved in outreach felt that they had development needs.

Experience within outreach is so rich and varied that there is a tremendous opportunity for work-based and experiential learning. This can be optimised through support systems or employing and evaluating strategies aimed at facilitating learning.

For practitioners there is a need to constantly balance the ability to act with the need to learn. This is especially true in a rapidly changing healthcare system. For those who are role models and leaders the need constantly to teach and share new knowledge and skills is also key.

Indicators of competence in this domain include an independent learner who identifies own needs, plans learning activity and records evidence of progress and competence. I have had the pleasure of working with a group of nurses who have exhibited this collectively. In this last section I want to share some further details about the group who helped developed these competencies and how they attempted to identify and meet their own learning and support needs.

LEARNING NETWORKS WITHIN OUTREACH

Critical care networks have changed not only the way critical care is delivered but also, fundamentally, the way practitioners collaborate, learn from each other and share best practice. There is a great potential for outreach practitioners to meet their learning needs more successfully if they collaborate within clinical networks. This has been demonstrated in the NTCCN (North Trent Critical Care Network) and some key features of this model are shared here.

The NTCCN was one of the first networks to be established. From the beginning there was a belief in the value of outreach. This resulted in pioneering work (Murch and Warren 2001) and the establishment of seven outreach teams within a 20-mile radius, including more than twenty outreach nurses, four consultant nurses and strong consultant anaesthetic support. The group of nurses began to meet early after establishing their teams with the objective of implementing educational programmes for acute ward staff. When this had been achieved there was a change in focus towards identifying and meeting the nurses' own learning needs.

Early work focused on identifying learning needs and the ideal competencies for the role. Following this plans were made to meet regularly and attempt to meet priority learning needs through a variety of activities including taught sessions. At one meeting nurses were asked to vote for the areas of highest priority. At the time (between 12 and 18 months after entering their new roles) the sessions thought to be highest priority were:

- systematic approach to patient assessment (history taking, physical assessment ordering and interpretation of diagnostic and laboratory tests);
- legal and professional issues in relation to the role of the outreach nurse;
- persuasion and influencing skills;
- audit;
- networks, NHS structures and funding;
- psychological/psychiatric disorders and intervention needs;
- publishing and presenting in professional forums.

As well as addressing these learning needs, other needs were identified that justified organising all day bimonthly meetings. Based on this a format for the meetings was agreed. This is presented in Box 11.11.

Box 11.11 Format of the bimonthly North Trent Critical Care Network outreach meetings

Format of each meeting

1. *Communications between teams* (e.g. introduction of new outreach nurses to the group, events, sharing of policies/protocols)
2. *Business items* (include issues of policy and principle, e.g. agreement to meet six times per year, roles and responsibilities of group members)

3. *Journal items* (e.g. sharing of recent reports, discussion articles, policies and political documents)
4. *Action learning* (e.g. sharing of experiences and case studies)
5. *Educational activity* (e.g. formal taught sessions by group members or guest speakers)

The meetings were a success with venues rotating around the seven hospitals and all teams taking responsibility for hosting and organising meetings. More than two years on, the meetings were still going strong though they were changed to a quarterly schedule. They have evolved to reflect the development and changing needs of the group. This would not have been possible without several core values being shared. These included:

- a willingness to share innovation, experiences and knowledge within the network, and beyond;
- a culture of innovation where the teams were open to alternative ways of doing things, of learning from experience and of using best evidence;
- a culture that recognised and valued the role of professional development in excellent nursing practice;
- a culture within which there was a willingness to share the tasks and responsibilities of bringing the teams together and moving forward as a network rather than as isolated groups.

The importance of these values cannot be overstated. They represent a major shift from the prevailing culture and inherent values of several years earlier. It would be a major omission not to acknowledge the role that documents such as *Comprehensive Critical Care* (DoH 2000) and clinical networks have played in this cultural change. However, it is also of paramount importance to acknowledge the contribution of the individuals who are part of that network and who have been driving forces in bringing professionals together. This is evidence of what can be achieved when nursing leadership is strengthened and the contribution that nurses make to care is valued, nurtured and supported.

POST-OUTREACH CAREER

In many ways outreach is liberating. It allows practitioners time to be innovative, to work autonomously as well as sharing the support of a small focused team. There is great potential to introduce new ways of doing things and developing new knowledge and skills. Outreach may act as a 'stepping stone' to many other levels of practice or to different career paths.

In the short time that outreach has existed staff have already moved on to other jobs. Examples of areas where people work after outreach include:

- return to or enter ICU or HDU;
- education – within a university setting or as a hospital-based teacher;
- practitioner/advanced practitioner – within critical care or in acute medicine or surgery;
- consultant practitioner – some outreach sisters/charge nurses have also gone on to work as consultant nurses;
- primary care.

The pathways to these other roles cannot be given full consideration here; however, there are some key points that are worth making. These are simple points but ones that are often neglected by practitioners considering a change.

- Moving on to another type of role or higher level of practice requires preparation in terms of your experience, knowledge, skills and qualifications. Investigate the role you aspire to thoroughly to maximise your chance of meeting the person specification.
- Investigate the role in order to decide whether it is for you: this might involve spending time shadowing someone who is already doing the job you aspire to.
- Ask someone in the role about their route into the job and how they prepared for it.
- Decide whether you really want to change jobs or just do something different for a short while or even re-negotiate your job plan or change your current role to incorporate work of a different type.
- Review your CV regularly – reflect on how your experience, skills, knowledge and qualifications fit with the person specification for the role. Plan how to address your areas of weakness.

CONCLUSION

The learning needs and processes of critical care outreach practitioners have received little consideration in the literature, though the need to address these has been acknowledged. Education for outreach practitioners has to reflect the context of the role and acknowledge the interventionist and educative supportive elements of outreach practice. Education needs also change over time for the individual practitioner and the team depending on the novelty of the practitioner to outreach or indeed the novelty of the team within the hospital. Early experiences of new teams highlight the need for abilities in diplomacy, service development and effective working within complex organisations.

While previous critical care unit experience may serve as a sound foundation for outreach practice, experiences from working outside of these units highlight the depth and breadth of learning required to fulfil the demands of the role. The chapter has not considered learning and development through academic routes and programmes of learning. Rather it has focused on learning in, from and through practice. With that focus it has presented preliminary work into the learning needs of a group of outreach nurses and has attempted to provide some practical strategies aimed at facilitating practice-based learning.

The experiences shared here highlighted an amount of disagreement over the competencies identified as being desirable for the role. This reflects the differing views and models of outreach even within a relatively small group who meet and share ideas regularly. The competencies discussed here are indicative rather than comprehensive, but they are seen as valid and meaningful in the context within which they were developed. Most importantly they have stimulated debate and critical thinking about them and the issues they raise for nursing. Such clarification exercises undertaken within collaborative and supportive networks of professionals can help set priorities for learning and strategies for meeting learning needs.

Critical care outreach is such a new role that there has been little time for career paths to be formalised and for the career options and development pathways to be refined. However, experiences to date suggest that far from being a narrow or limiting role, outreach offers great opportunities for learning and development in many domains of professional practice. The career options open to the critical care nurse who has experience in outreach can only be enhanced compared to those who work within the 'walls' of critical care.

A FINAL WORD ON LEARNING

There is a theme within outreach that is a feature of adult learning more generally. That is moving 'out of the comfort zone' is frustrating and can be emotionally draining. But the soul searching and deep reflection that result are a powerful way of learning. Learning that is of great value does not come without significant effort and emotional engagement.

REFERENCES

Anderson K, Atkinson D, McBride J, Moorse S, Smith S (2002) Setting up an outreach team in the UK. *Connect: Critical Care Nursing in Europe* 2(1): 8–12.
Brookfield SD (1995) *Becoming a Critically Reflective Teacher.* San Francisco: Jossey-Bass.

Charters A (2000) Role modelling as a teaching method. *Emergency Nurse* 7(10): 25–9.

Coombs M (2002) Critical care outreach: short-term measure or long-term solution? *Nursing in Critical Care* 7(3): 109–10.

Coombs M, Moorse SE (2002) Physical assessment skills: a developing dimension of clinical nursing practice. *Intensive and Critical Care Nursing* 18(4): 200–10.

Davies E (1993) Clinical role modelling: uncovering hidden knowledge. *Journal of Advanced Nursing.* 18(4): 627–36.

Department of Health (1999) *Agenda for Change: Modernising the NHS Pay System.* London: Department of Health.

Department of Health (2000) *Comprehensive Critical Care: A Review of Adult Critical Care Services.* London: Department of Health.

Department of Health (2001) *The Nursing Contribution to Comprehensive Critical Care.* London: Department of Health.

Department of Health (2004) *NHS Knowledge and Skills Framework Handbook.* London: Department of Health.

Flannagan J, Baldwin S, Clarke E (2000) Work-based learning as a means of developing and assessing nursing competence. *Journal of Clinical Nursing* 9: 360–8.

Fulbrook P (2004) Realizing advanced nursing practice through reflection. Editorial. *Nursing in Critical Care* 9(6): 255–6.

Milligan F (1998) Defining and assessing competence, the distraction of outcomes and the importance of educational process. *Nurse Education Today* 18: 273–80.

Modernisation Agency (2003) *The National Outreach Report 2003: Critical Care Outreach 2003 – Progress in Developing Services.* London: Department of Health and Modernisation Agency.

Murch P, Warren K (2001) Developing the role of the critical care liaison nurse. *Nursing in Critical Care* 6(5): 221–5.

Scholes J, Endacott R (2003) The practice competency gap: challenges that impede the introduction of national core competencies. *Nursing in Critical Care* 8(2): 68–77.

Schon DA (1987) *Educating the Reflective Practitioner.* San Francisco: Jossey-Bass.

Younker J (2002) Outreach: are we speaking the same language? Editorial. *Nursing in Critical Care.* 7(2): 56–8.

V Developing and Evaluating Critical Care Outreach

12 Managing change in critical care: a toolkit for practice

NICOLA PLATTS AND SUE SHEPHERD

In writing this chapter we aim to provide you with a toolkit that will help you examine your current practices, introduce changes and improve services. The chapter does not aim to be theoretical, but provides practical information on how to implement change using a set of clearly explained tools and techniques, and where possible we have used examples relating to critical care outreach. There are a lot of texts written on change management and process redesign and we have included some of these for reference at the end of the chapter should you wish to explore the theory further.

The framework outlined in this chapter is based on *The Model for Improvement* (Langley et al. 1996) as illustrated in Figure 12.1 which has been adopted by the NHS in England and Wales. We have collated, tried, tested and developed the tools and techniques over the last three years in critical care units in hospitals within the Trent and South Yorkshire regions as part of the National Health Service (NHS) Modernisation Agency (MA) National Critical Care Service Improvement Programme. In doing this we have used ideas, tools and tips provided by other colleagues working in a number of MA programmes and acknowledge their willingness and openness in sharing their work, some of which we will share with you throughout this chapter.

We recognise that one approach does not fit all projects, so the information provided represents a 'toolbox' of materials that enables you to 'pick and mix' tools and ideas to suit your own situation. Through *The Model for Improvement* we are providing you with a structured framework to enable you to undertake change projects. However on occasion you might find it more useful to move backwards and forwards through the model, checking or changing what you are doing at each stage and there is no problem with this. What we are offering you is a set of tools and techniques for you to use if and when you think they will be useful.

We recognise the complexity of critical care outreach and acknowledge that in order for you to implement any changes you might have to involve a large number of people from many different departments. Many of the change

Critical Care Outreach. Edited by Lee Cutler and Wayne Robson.
Copyright 2006 by John Wiley & Sons Ltd.

programmes that have been undertaken in the NHS over the last few years have faced similar challenges and by using *The Model for Improvement* they have succeeded in implementing changes and have demonstrated a number of improvements. We hope that you will have the same success.

THE MODEL FOR IMPROVEMENT

You can be involved in improving health services by exploring and questioning the way care is delivered to your patients. Many different approaches to the way we change services have been tried and tested in the NHS over the years. Redesign is one approach, which is defined as 'thinking through the best process to achieve fast and effective care from the patient perspective' (Iles and Sutherland 2001). *The Model for Improvement* serves as a guide for redesign, reminding the change team to fully understand the process and the real problems before finding a solution, involve key staff and use scientific methods to guide decisions. As well as a guide, the model serves as a common approach and language for improvement, making it easier for people from different disciplines and backgrounds to work together (Plesk 1999).

The key feature of *The Model for Improvement* is to think small and learn fast. Small changes made now can have a big effect, which in turn will hopefully result in a more efficient use of limited resources. For example, think of some of the problems associated with caring for tracheostomy patients on discharge from critical care to the wards. By the critical care team providing essential tracheostomy equipment to the ward when the patient is discharged, delays in finding equipment will be eliminated. This is a simple change that will have a big effect in improving the care of the patient and reducing time, effort and frustrations for ward and critical care staff.

Donald Berwick, President and Chief Executive Officer of the Institute of Healthcare Improvement in the USA, stated, 'because risk, anxiety, and costs are so heavily concentrated in the intensive care environment, the opportunities for improvement in the ICU are also the greatest' (Rainey et al. 1998). We have been using the model with staff in the critical care environment over the last few years and have found it an effective method for introducing changes.

So, why is the model useful and how does it help? One of the biggest issues is that most people try and come up with a solution to a problem without actually knowing what the *real* problem is. Using *The Model for Improvement* helps you examine what is happening on a day-to-day basis and identify the root cause of the problem. Although at first it might seem like this is slowing things down, we have found that spending time identifying the real problem, getting everyone involved, and having an effective action plan generally saves time in the long run and more importantly can make a real difference to patient care.

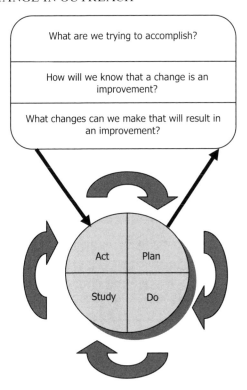

Figure 12.1 Model for Improvement. Reprinted from www.IHI.org with permission of the Institute for Healthcare Improvement (IHI) © 2005.

The model requires you to think about what you are trying to accomplish (aim), how you will know that a change that you implement is effecting an improvement (measurable outcomes) and what changes you can make that will result in an improvement (change ideas). It allows a trial and learning approach to change ideas with change being measured continuously. This means that as a team you can find out what is working and what is not and make changes as necessary. Some changes will be made following the initial change idea, but often multiple changes may be needed before the desired aim is achieved.

The Plan, Do, Study, Act (PDSA) cycle adopts an incremental evidence based approach to change where new ideas are piloted on small samples initially. Each test cycle is planned (plan) then carried out (do). The results are then evaluated (study) prior to further testing or implementation (act). The PDSA approach encourages you as an individual and a team to reflect critically on your successes and failures. Use of PDSA cycles is a way of testing an idea by putting a change into effect on a temporary basis and learning from its potential impact.

STARTING YOUR CHANGE PROJECT

So where do you start? The first thing that usually happens is that you or a colleague has a gut feeling that things aren't quite right and could be better. So where do you go from here, how do you move from 'me' to 'we' and have the confidence to try out an idea? You need to think about who will be affected and involve all the key people at an early stage so that everyone is clear about the reason or need for the change. If you are leading the project, it's useful if you can help everyone to understand the current problems, why the change is necessary, what could happen if things don't change and what could happen if things do change. Using the model for improvement, the first question is 'What are we trying to accomplish?'

Box 12.1 What are we trying to accomplish?

• What is it you want to do?
• What do you hope to see as a result of the change?
• Why do you think it will make a difference?

WHAT ARE WE TRYING TO ACCOMPLISH?

This is about developing your initial hunch or idea that there is a problem or issue and analysing it further which is particularly useful if you need to convince others of the need to change. Thinking about what you want to accomplish also allows you to take time to think through how things could really be in order to promote a positive and compelling vision. Once you've thought through the initial idea for the project you need to think a bit more about the real issue and ask the questions posed in Box 12.2.

Box 12.2 What are we trying to accomplish?

• Why focus on this issue?
• How do you think patients, carers or relatives and staff may benefit?
• What is happening now? (What, when, where, how often?)
• What will happen if things don't improve?
• What are the factors that are hindering you from moving forward?

Using the responses to the questions in Box 12.2 will help you to develop an aim statement.

DEVELOPING AN AIM STATEMENT

An aim statement helps you to clearly define the purpose of your project and importantly the outcomes you hope to achieve. It also helps you focus on a specific group of patients. Once you have developed your aim statement you need to make sure that you communicate it to everyone involved. When you come to identify changes to the process you can keep checking that they contribute to the intended aim of the project. If they do, then you are more likely to see improvements, if your ideas move further away from the aim of your project you might need to reassess what you are doing. You can keep revisiting your aim and refining it as necessary throughout the project to ensure it remains appropriate.

When writing an aim statement it is useful to consider the points in Box 12.3.

Box 12.3 Developing an aim statement

- What you hope to improve, e.g. access, patient experience, and reduction in time
- The group of patients you will be including, e.g. emergency, elective, surgical
- Where the process will start and end, in other words, the scope of the project, e.g. from the time the patient is ready for discharge from the critical care unit to the time they are admitted to the ward

---

Table 12.1 gives a few examples of an aim statement.

So now you have thought through the real issues, and identified a project aim, you are ready to move on to the next stage of the framework and think about how you will demonstrate that any changes you make will be an improvement.

Table 12.1 Aim statement

To improve the care of all patients who have a percutaneous or surgical tracheostomy by standardising and optimising their care and management in ICU and on the wards.

To improve patient outcome by decreasing the time it takes to wean patients from the ventilator.

To reduce the time taken for postoperative orthopaedic patients who become hypotensive to receive the first bolus of fluid.

HOW WILL WE KNOW THAT CHANGE IS AN IMPROVEMENT?

It's at this point that you need to start thinking about what you can measure in order to show progress in relation to the aim of the project; in other words collect some data to support your need for change. Often there is a lack of agreement in the group of what the nature of the problem is or even if there is a problem. Having data can help reduce the effects that strong opinions from colleagues can have on a project and more easily demonstrates the need for change. What you need to agree is a few specific measures linked to the project that will help to show if improvements are being made.

When thinking about the changes you plan to make or where you might want to try and make things better, it's important that you think about who will be affected by the change and where possible make the new way attractive to each person by linking it to something that appeals to them, e.g. best for the patient, reducing paperwork or fewer steps in a process. Make sure you communicate these advantages if the change makes them possible. People are much more likely to adopt the changes if they can see the benefit that appeals to them, particularly where the change is likely to create more time either for themselves or for the system. So when you are thinking about your measures and what data you will need to collect, think about the points raised in Box 12.4.

Box 12.4 Data collection and measurement

- Do you already have any data that you can use to support the need for change?
- If not, what data can you collect to support the need for change?
- Do you have any patient stories or useful anecdotes of experiences to support the need for change?
- If successful/unsuccessful, what would you expect to see?
- What is a sensible target?

In addition to the above, remember to keep in mind what it is you are trying to accomplish. The measures you select do not need to be difficult or complex, in fact the simpler the better. Remember that the aim is to make improvements and not get bogged down with obtaining perfect data. The areas we work in are very complex with external events happening all the time that affect the results of our projects. Researchers try hard to minimise the impact of external changes in their experiments by ensuring that control and intervention groups are matched as closely as possible for example, by age, gender and severity of disease. They also use large sample sizes to be able to get statistical evidence that the intervention they have made is successful. This is because research is about providing us with certainty that a new intervention, a new medication for example, is the best or better than the alternative for a specific group of patients wherever they are treated. By contrast you just want to be certain that best practice is being adopted in a way that is appropriate to your local situation. You only need to be comfortable that the data you have collected is sufficient to enable you to be clear about the effect your changes have had and what steps you need to take next. Most importantly your choice of measures should be influenced by who will use the data and what they will use it for.

What you need to collect are small representative samples that can be built into your daily work, for example, if it would be too time-consuming and costly to collect data on all patients then collect data on every tenth patient or for all respiratory patients each Thursday. Collecting sample data in this way ensures that data quality is maintained.

When thinking about your measures remember to start small, for example, your aim may be to reduce the number of cancelled operations due to the lack of a critical care bed. You may have identified a number of ideas for improvement, for example, improving access to the high dependency unit by establishing standard discharge criteria and enabling nursing staff to start the discharge process thereby reducing the delay in discharging patients who are fit for discharge to the ward. The team could not expect to impact on the overall aim straight away so to keep the momentum of the project going the team may measure the time from patient identified as fit to discharge to the time they left the unit. This measure is appropriate to the scale of the change being tested as well as monitoring the cancelled elective rate throughout the project.

If you have previously been involved in projects, particularly service improvement projects, think about the sorts of issues that have affected these projects. We either collect lots and lots of data and have difficulty interpreting it, which results in few changes, or we make lots of changes and do not measure the result so we are unable demonstrate the impact our work has had. In our experience, this last issue is particularly pertinent in that we have undertaken many projects with lots of staff in critical care and still we have difficulty collecting the data for measurement. However, making a particular effort in this area really does pay off because once you have the data displayed in an appropriate format it really does help to demonstrate to your colleagues where you have made improvements or changes, or in fact where it has little effect which is just as important for subsequent change ideas. We

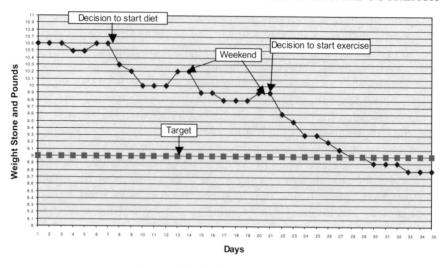

Figure 12.2 Weight loss run chart.

have found that run charts are a really effective way of displaying the measurement data for these projects (see Figure 12.2). Run charts show trends in improvement and enable you to slowly build evidence to demonstrate whether the change has made a difference or not. Once the data is displayed in this way and shared with the rest of the team you can easily see whether the change is making things better or worse and this can be a real motivator for the team members and help to build the project further. It is possible to apply some simple statistics to run charts to help you understand the variations you see in your data and prove that your change has made an impact. These graphs, called control charts, are outside the remit of this chapter and are covered in detail elsewhere (Goal/QPC 1995; Plesk 1999). You may find it helpful to seek out the advice of someone who has knowledge of 'statistical process control' if you want to construct a control chart from your data but a run chart is often all that is needed to visually display the result of your changes.

DATA COLLECTION AND MEASUREMENT CHECKLIST TOOLBOX

The key to successful data collection is primarily being clear about the intended use of the data and how you will analyse it once it is collected (Table 12.2 and Box 12.5).

Table 12.2 Use of data

1. What question do you need to answer – why are you collecting this data?	For example, has the improvement effort to standardise the care of patients on mechanical ventilation reduced the time patients spend on mechanical ventilation?
2. What kind of data will you need to collect?	To answer the question above the team could measure the time patients spend on the ventilator in days or in hours. If the data was collected in hours it would be easier to see variations and small improvements. Consider having measures in place to check that changes being made to one part of the system are not causing problems in other parts of the system. For example, reducing time patients spend on the ventilator make sure that reintubation rates are not increasing.
3. How do you intend to display the data once it has been collected?	Draw out a mock table or graph using made up numbers as if the pilot project had been successful or unsuccessful. Would the data displayed in this way answer your question? Run charts are a recommended way to display data showing changes over time.

Box 12.5 Developing your data collection plan

- Who will collect the data?
- What data will be collected?
- When will the data be collected?
- Where will the data be collected?
- How will the data be collected?
- How much data will be collected?
- Test the method devised in the above questions with a few people who will actually be collecting the data and incorporate their ideas for improving the process.
- Teach all the data collectors how to collect the data correctly.
- Record what went wrong during the data collection so that lessons can be learnt.
- Check the data as it comes in for completeness and accuracy and correct as soon as possible.
- Provide feedback in a timely way, for example, post the graph up on the unit, discuss at regular meetings.

Adapted from Simple Data Collection Planning, Information Gathering Tools, www.QualityHealthCare.org

So now you have started to think about how you can measure the change, you need to move on to the next stage of the model and start to think about where you can make some changes to get you nearer to where you want to be.

WHAT CHANGES CAN WE MAKE THAT WILL RESULT IN AN IMPROVEMENT?

In order that you have a clear understanding of where you can make changes that might have some sort of impact and make an improvement, you need to be sure that you have a really clear understanding of the process you are trying to change. Sometimes you might 'think' that you know what is happening and where you can make changes, but without really looking in detail at the process there is a danger that you might in fact make inappropriate changes to the wrong part of the process.

The challenge here is to analyse fully what is happening now before trying to come up with potential solutions. By spending time early on defining the real problem it is more likely that the solutions you test will be the successful ones. This avoids the risk of falling into the trap of trying to 'sell a solution' to a team of people who do not really understand the problem you are trying to solve. This is an opportunity to get others involved, helping them to identify for themselves the need for change and generate their own ideas for what changes could be made. One of the potential dangers is that the project is hijacked by the person/people with the loudest voices or the self-appointed leaders who have a strong opinion of what the solutions are. Facilitated sessions using tools such as process mapping are an excellent way to create a safe environment for people to question the current situation and see it from another point of view such as from the point of view of other members of staff, patients or their carers. So what is process mapping and what are the benefits?

PROCESS MAPPING

A process is a series of connected steps or actions to achieve an outcome (DoH 2005). Most things we do are a process – shopping, mowing the lawn, making a cup of coffee. Mapping a process enables you to identify what happens in reality and provides you with a visual picture of the complexities involved (Figure 12.3).

It is a method that allows all the people closest to the process to come together and clearly identify how the work actually gets done. It is often the first time everyone has seen the process clearly displayed from start to finish and people are often surprised by how many steps are involved in the process,

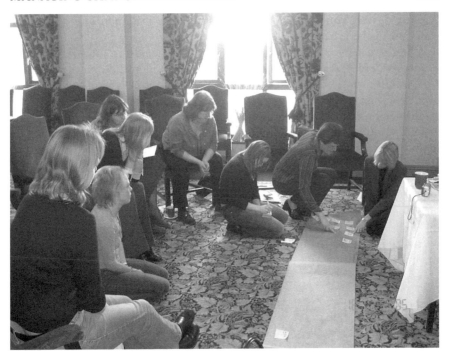

Figure 12.3 Photo of process mapping session (Mid Trent Critical Care Network).

as well as by who does what where. Process mapping is a useful tool because it focuses everyone on finding the real source of the problem in the process. This is where the real involving and engaging comes into the project because everyone has an opportunity to be involved in building up the picture. People start to become enthusiastic and own the issues and together start to develop an action plan, a clear way forward for the project. Once complete the process allows you to question what is really happening, who does what, where and when and why we do things in a certain way. In other words it provides an ideal opportunity to fully analyse the current situation. Process mapping helps you to clearly identify what is happening for the majority of the time and helps you focus on key issues in the way the service is delivered. Working together in this way enables you to focus on the patient and is a way of bringing other teams and services together from across the organisation. It enables you to see why changes are necessary and is a really effective way of drawing out some creative and brilliant ideas. Process mapping can be undertaken at different levels. You might often start with a high level map, which gives an overview of the process (Figure 12.4).

When you have analysed the map you may decide to map part of the process where particular issues or problems are identified in more detail. This might mean that you need to involve different people in the mapping process in order to really understand what is happening. At this stage you might decide to follow a patient through the process and in doing this you can start to collect some data on how long each step is taking, which will in fact give you some baseline data that you can use for demonstrating the change.

Once you have mapped a process you can start to ask questions to help you identify areas where improvements could be made (Box 12.6). We have listed quite a lot of questions here and they may not always all be relevant, depending on how detailed your process map is, the more detailed the more you may want to move down the list of questions, or if you prefer, just pick and choose the ones relevant for you on the day.

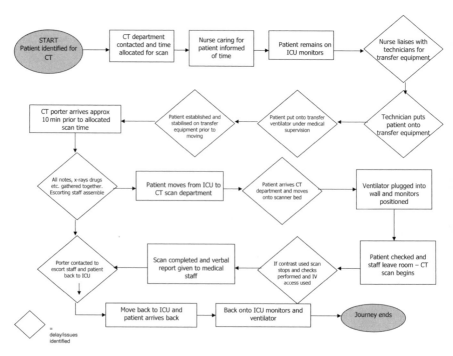

Figure 12.4 Example of a high level process map: mapping the patient's journey to CT scan (Mid Trent Critical Care Network).

Box 12.6 Analysing the process

- How many steps are in your process?
- How many steps in the process are adding no value to the patient journey?
- Where are the delays or blockages in the system?
- Are any vital steps missing?
- What concerns or issues do patients have?
- What concerns or issues do relatives/carers have?
- What concerns or issues do staff have?
- Purpose – why does this step occur here in the process?
- Place – should it be done there?
- Sequence – is this the best order of events?
- People – should this person be doing it?
- Method – is there a better way?
- Is the right person doing the right thing at the right time?
- Where is the biggest problem?
- Any change ideas?
- What changes can we make to the way that we deliver the service?
- Who are the key stakeholders and how can we engage them?

Drawing up an action plan at the end of the mapping session allows you to have a clearly defined plan for taking the project forward. In addition it allows you to seek the views of people who are involved in the process who may not have been present on the day (Box 12.7).

Box 12.7 Developing an action plan

- Which parts of process need to mapped in more detail? How will this be arranged?
- Who should communicate to people not here?
- When and how are you going to generate ideas to test once the process is fully understood?
- Make sure everyone clearly understands who will do what, by when?

KEEPING EVERYONE ON BOARD

The steps we have outlined above help you to put together a sound case for change. However, although process mapping gives everyone the opportunity to be involved it's important to recognise that some people may not fully participate in the mapping session for a variety of different reasons. Some people may not feel comfortable with the people around the table. There may be one or more dominant people in the group who give little opportunity for other people to express their opinions. People may feel shy and not confident to express their own opinions. In our experience, this is particularly true of more junior nursing staff who may not feel confident to express their opinion in front of a room full of more experienced senior staff. Other people might not fully understand what the group is trying to achieve or do not see the issue as a priority in their own agenda. If you are facilitating a mapping session (Bens 2000), you need to provide the opportunity for everyone to be involved and let everyone know that their opinion is valued. Think about what the change means for the individuals and help them see the benefits for them as individuals as well as the bigger benefits to the service. Make sure that everyone has a clear understanding of what is expected of them and help them to see how their bit fits into the overall picture. Some people may be concerned about the amount of time they may be expected to spend in project meetings. Help them to see that once the changes are in place this should mean less frustration or a better process, which might in fact save them time in the long run. This does of course depend on what process is being examined.

In our experience, if you involve people in mapping the process they are likely to become more interested and start to become engaged in the project (Figure 12.5). There are no easy shortcuts to the buy in stage, the best approach is to try and pull people with you rather than trying to push them. Bringing everyone together in order to map the process also gives you an opportunity to examine the relationships between the people involved in the process and enables you to identify where these relationships may need to be developed further in order to allow the change to take place. You may need to have individual meetings with key stakeholders to find out what they feel about the proposed change and what is preventing them from participating fully and this will help you to understand what you can do to help them work with you to effect the change. It might help if at each meeting you revisit the aim statement, making sure everyone is clear about the aim of the project, making adjustments as necessary. Regular meetings provide a good opportunity to share ideas and share outcomes from any work that has already been undertaken in the project, which should help the group to see that changes are being made and that things are improving. You might want to choose a few simple measures to monitor how you are progressing and review these measures at each meeting. In addition you need to agree any tasks and responsibilities for specific members of the group in order to take the project forward and you might find it helpful to consider the points raised in Box 12.8.

Box 12.8 Keeping everyone on board

- Agree on the main cause of the problem or issue and agree what change you are going to test which might give the best improvement.
- Who is doing – or will do – what, when and where?
- Identify a senior member of staff (clinical director, matron) who believes in what you are trying to do and has authority over all the areas affected by the change who can use their authority to overcome any barriers you may encounter.
- What you need the above person to do is to clearly demonstrate the importance of the change and their commitment to it.
- Identify those colleagues who others look to for advice on this topic, or when learning about new ways of doing things, are supportive of your project and can help get others on board.
- What you need the above person to do to influence their colleagues?
- Agree how you will report progress of the project to all interested parties?

So now you have mapped and analysed the process. You have completed the first three stages in the model and you should have identified all the possible causes of any problems. This should have given you some idea of where you can make changes that will improve the system or process. You need now to decide which change you want to test out first. Some things will be easier to try out and you can just get on and test these. However, other change ideas may need a bit more thought and planning before you can test them. Once you have reached this stage you are ready to test out the changes using the PDSA cycle.

TESTING OUT THE CHANGES

At this stage the change idea may be just that, an idea or a theory. You might be uncertain about the impact the change could have. You might have consensus from others in your own profession that the change will bring about an improvement but are experiencing doubts from colleagues in other professions. The PDSA cycle enables you to test out your ideas before implementing any changes and provides you with a way forward, step by step. It helps you to keep things moving and prevents you getting stuck in a long planning stage. So where do you start?

Steps in mapping a process:

The aim of this tool is to help guide you through the steps involved in mapping a
patient journey, however there is no right or wrong way to process map, you can adapt
the tool to suit your circumstances.

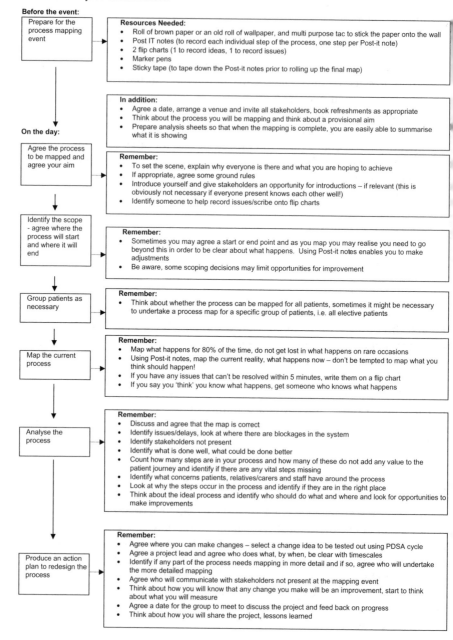

Before the event:

Prepare for the process mapping event

Resources Needed:
- Roll of brown paper or an old roll of wallpaper, and multi purpose tac to stick the paper onto the wall
- Post IT notes (to record each individual step of the process, one step per Post-it note)
- 2 flip charts (1 to record ideas, 1 to record issues)
- Marker pens
- Sticky tape (to tape down the Post-it notes prior to rolling up the final map)

In addition:
- Agree a date, arrange a venue and invite all stakeholders, book refreshments as appropriate
- Think about the process you will be mapping and think about a provisional aim
- Prepare analysis sheets so that when the mapping is complete, you are easily able to summarise what it is showing

On the day:

Agree the process to be mapped and agree your aim

Remember:
- To set the scene, explain why everyone is there and what you are hoping to achieve
- If appropriate, agree some ground rules
- Introduce yourself and give stakeholders an opportunity for introductions – if relevant (this is obviously not necessary if everyone present knows each other well!)
- Identify someone to help record issues/scribe onto flip charts

Identify the scope - agree where the process will start and where it will end

Remember:
- Sometimes you may agree a start or end point and as you map you may realise you need to go beyond this in order to be clear about what happens. Using Post-it notes enables you to make adjustments
- Be aware, some scoping decisions may limit opportunities for improvement

Group patients as necessary

Remember:
- Think about whether the process can be mapped for all patients, sometimes it might be necessary to undertake a process map for a specific group of patients, i.e. all elective patients

Map the current process

Remember:
- Map what happens for 80% of the time, do not get lost in what happens on rare occasions
- Using Post-it notes, map the current reality, what happens now – don't be tempted to map what you think should happen!
- If you have any issues that can't be resolved within 5 minutes, write them on a flip chart
- If you say you 'think' you know what happens, get someone who knows what happens

Analyse the process

Remember:
- Discuss and agree that the map is correct
- Identify issues/delays, look at where there are blockages in the system
- Identify stakeholders not present
- Identify what is done well, what could be done better
- Count how many steps are in your process and how many of these do not add any value to the patient journey and identify if there are any vital steps missing
- Identify what concerns patients, relatives/carers and staff have around the process
- Look at why the steps occur in the process and identify if they are in the right place
- Think about the ideal process and identify who should do what and where and look for opportunities to make improvements

Produce an action plan to redesign the process

Remember:
- Agree where you can make changes – select a change idea to be tested out using PDSA cycle
- Agree a project lead and agree who does what, by when, be clear with timescales
- Identify if any part of the process needs mapping in more detail and if so, agree who will undertake the more detailed mapping
- Agree who will communicate with stakeholders not present at the mapping event
- Think about how you will know that any change you make will be an improvement, start to think about what you will measure
- Agree a date for the group to meet to discuss the project and feed back on progress
- Think about how you will share the project, lessons learned

Figure 12.5 Steps in mapping a process.

Plan

When you start your project look for changes that will have the most impact but are relatively easy to introduce. Our advice would be that it's probably best not to start with a change that requires a long lead in time or requires you to get full committee approval first as this might slow the process down and, in doing so, people might lose interest in the project before you've had a chance to test any change ideas. For your first change idea it may be best to work with people who want to work with you, people who are supportive of the change. So in selecting your patients, you might decide to test the change on the next two patients discharged from ICU who are under consultant X. Remember, this model is designed to enable you to test changes on a small scale. So this does not mean that you need to undertake grand scale research or audit. You can test out the change with one or two patients on the unit or ward, with every third patient on a ventilator or the next three patients to be discharged from HDU, whatever is relevant to your proposed change idea.

Think about what the process mapping showed you and the aim of your project. The questions in Box 12.9 will help you to plan your first change cycle.

Box 12.9 PDSA cycle – Plan

- What is the objective of the first change you are going to test?
- What exactly will you do?
- Who will be involved?
- Where will it take place?
- When will it take place, over what period of time?
- How will you know the change has been a success?
- What data/information do you need to collect?
- What do you predict could happen?
- What could go wrong?
- What organisational barriers could you run into?
- Are there any human resource issues?
- What may prevent members of the team doing the task?
- What may change to alter priorities?
- What actions could you take to overcome some of the anticipated problems if they arise?

So, now you have planned your first change, you are ready to carry out the plan and move on to the next stage of the testing cycle.

Do

Try to follow the plan as it was designed but document any necessary changes to the plan with the reasons why the change had to take place so that you can learn from the process. As you undertake the change, also make a note of any problems or issues or any unexpected outcomes or observations. As you carry out the change, continue to collect data to measure your progress. The PDSA approach offers a safety net because the reflection and measurement is done close to where the action happens so any failure should not cause harm, i.e. reducing any inherent risk. The added advantage is that by recording any unpredicted changes you can then look at these in more detail and if necessary test these changes for improvement in the next change cycle. The next stage, the Study part of the cycle is where we analyse the Do stage. Did we do what we planned to do and did it have the positive impact we predicted it would have?

Study

This is your opportunity to reflect on the changes you have made and analyse the effects of the change. This will help you in deciding whether to implement the change at the Act stage or not depending on whether the change resulted in an improvement or not. At this stage you also need to complete the analysis of the data and compare what the data is showing you to your initial thoughts and predictions. After making a change the team should ask the questions in Box 12.10.

Box 12.10 PDSA cycle – Study

- What were the results?
- Did we expect this to happen?
- What have we learned?
- What was good about this change?
- What was bad about this change?

Once you have completed your test of the change you are ready to examine the effects and decide what you are going to do. This moves you on to the final stage of the test cycle, the Act.

Act

So now you have planned and undertaken your change idea and examined the effects, you need to look at what changes you are going to make or whether there is something else that you wish to test out which will move you on to the next test cycle. If the change has had a positive effect then you may decide to implement the change. If it has not, then you might decide to abandon the change idea. At this stage it's wise to consider whether there is anything else that can be done or tested in another test cycle. If there really isn't anything that you think will make any improvements, then you might decide at this stage to complete the project, reflect on what has been learned and share the learning with the group. You must not at any stage be concerned about completing an improvement project, if it has run its course then the wisest thing you can do is to stop. On the other hand, if your change idea is showing some sort of improvement then you might want to consider the questions in Box 12.11.

Box 12.11 PDSA – Act

- What shall we do next?
- What further issues or problems are likely to require action?
- What future issues or problems are likely to occur?
- What can we plan to do to reduce the impact of these?
- Who is responsible for each action?

You are now ready to move back to the Plan, Do, Study, Act cycle to test out your new idea.

SPREADING AND MAINTAINING THE SUCCESSES

You have tested out your initial change ideas on a small scale, some ideas may have been abandoned but hopefully some will have proven to be successful in achieving your aim. How do you ensure that more of your colleagues are aware of the benefit of these changes and convince them to adopt them? Suggested reading material on this subject is included at the end of this chapter (Fraser 2002; Berwick 2003).

You need to ensure that when you are explaining the change or project to your colleagues, you identify all the changes and improvements and share with them why the project has improved the current way of doing things, in particular how it will help them and their patients. Use your data to illustrate the point. If you are giving information to staff in a different profession to your own you may find it useful to have it checked by someone in the same profession as your target audience. Simple differences in language used may turn some people off so try and see things from their perspective, or try and help everyone to see it from the patients' perspective.

People are reluctant to introduce changes when they are uncertain whether they are going to get a positive result or they are concerned about the risks. Make the results of your trial visible and share it in a way that is easy to interpret, for example, your run chart. It is also of value to share *The Model for Improvement* so that you can explain that the change can continue to be tested on a small scale without being implemented everywhere straightaway and that if the person you are talking to would prefer they could see others trial the change first so that they can see what results they achieve and what time and effort the changes would require. Finally, make it clear what the first steps would be if they decided to test the change.

We know from experience that this stage, maintaining the momentum of the project, is hard. Other changes such as an increase or decrease in case load or changes to the processes carried out by other departments that impact on critical care are just some of the other challenges to the sustainability of your project. There are issues of keeping everyone informed amid frequent staff changes in some organisations and amid an array of external priorities. In keeping everyone informed it is best to use a variety of different communication methods and use more than one method at one time; for example, use the broad brush approach such as flyers, newsletters, posters and reports as well as the more personal approach such as meetings with key people and telephone conversations. Also, interactive events such as workshops or seminars are a good way to share the details and get feedback, as are presentations at local events or conferences (Fraser 2002).

So now you have hopefully completed your project and have seen some real improvements for the benefits of patients, staff and/or carers. Remember to share your learning and experience and congratulate your team on their success. The changes you introduce may be the best for the process as it is at this time but as the service continues to evolve it is important to revisit your process map now and again and check your data to see if the old problems have recurred or if there are other issues arising. In this way you can continue to make changes to ensure that the improvements you have seen are maintained.

CASE STUDY

IMPROVING PATIENT FLUID MANAGEMENT POST OPERATIVELY

Example using The Model for Improvement – for illustration only

What are we trying to accomplish?

The outreach team felt that they were frequently being bleeped by ward staff for advice on the care of postoperative patients needing fluid. On review of the data they found 26% of calls from the wards were for this group of patients. They had a hunch that patients were waiting an inappropriately long time to receive a fluid, which could lead to patients going on to develop more serious complications. They agreed that they wanted to ensure that all post-operative patients got the same standard of care and initially they decided to limit their focus to orthopaedic postoperative patients. The team agreed that the aim of their project would be:

To reduce the time taken for postoperative orthopaedic patients who become hypotensive to receive the first bolus of fluid.

How will we know that change is an improvement?

The team decided to collect some simple data on the next 15 postoperative patients they were notified of to see if the problem was as they anticipated. The measure they chose was the time from nurse assessment of patient hypotension to the time the patient received a bolus of fluid. The run chart (Figure 12.6) shows the simple baseline data they collected. They found that the time between the nurse assessment of hypotension and the time the patient received a bolus of fluid ranged from 0 to 220 minutes (median 40 minutes).

What changes can we make that will lead to an improvement?

The critical care outreach team were alarmed at the data they collected and after discussion with colleagues in orthopaedics they decided that something needed to be done. A meeting was held to process map what was happening and find out what changes could be made. Three consultant orthopaedic surgeons, two nurse practitioners from general surgery, a consultant anaesthetist from ICU and the head of pharmacy attended the meeting facilitated by the

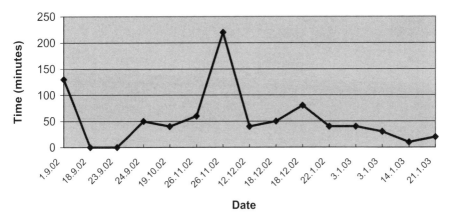

Figure 12.6 Fluid management baseline run chart.

outreach team. They agreed that the aim would be to reduce the time taken for postoperative orthopaedic patients to receive fluid to ten minutes or less from the time their need for fluid was recognised. The group agreed that the process they would map started with the arrival of the patient on the ward from theatre and ended with the administration of fluid. The finished process map is shown in Figure 12.7.

Process map analysis

Once the process map was complete, the group analysed the map and identified the following issues.

- Insufficient handover information from theatres means that ward nurses have to search patient notes for information on the patient's normal physical state and details of the fluid given in theatre, which delayed the proper assessment of the patient by the ward staff.
- Variation between nursing staff on the indicators used to recognise fluid needed which could delay identification of need for fluid when the patient was on the ward.
- Delay in contacting the surgical team for instructions, particularly after 5:00 pm and at weekends when staff cover is lower.
- Variation in the instructions given by the medical team to the ward nurses depending on time of day or day of the week.

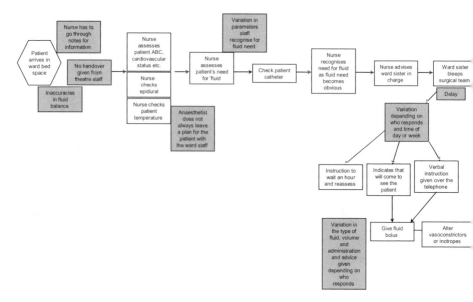

Figure 12.7 Fluid process map.

- Variation in the type of fluid and method of administration depending on the preference of the member of medical staff administering the treatment.

The group identified the following change ideas:

1. Introduce a handover checklist to ensure that vital information was communicated between the theatre and the ward staff.
2. Develop and trial a standard fluid management guideline to ensure: the same method was used to recognise the need for fluid, the same type of fluid and method of administration was agreed and assessment was carried out at regular intervals.
3. Enable nursing staff on the wards to administer fluid under the guideline.

The group agreed that the fluid management guideline was likely to give the best improvement in achieving their aim to reduce the time taken for post-operative patients to receive the first bolus of fluid. At the end of the meeting the following action plan was agreed.

Plan: Draft fluid management guideline to be drawn up by the nurse practitioners, the nurse consultant from ICU and the head of pharmacy and circulated to orthopaedic and critical care staff for comment by an agreed date. Presentation to be made by the nurse consultant to all orthopaedic consultants at their next forum meeting to discuss the current problems and why the team wanted to test the guideline. The project team met again to discuss progress.

Do: The fluid management guideline was drawn up and circulated by the agreed deadline. The process map and the draft guideline was presented by the nurse consultant at the orthopaedic directorate consultant forum as planned.

Study: Two of the orthopaedic consultants agreed for their patients to be included in a trial. The team felt that the presentation to the orthopaedic consultant forum went well although they agreed that at future meetings they would invite the clinical director for surgical services who was supportive of their project to introduce the project as this might have engaged more of the consultants.

Act: Next Tuesday morning trial the guideline on the first three patients (managed by the surgeons who have agreed to the trial) to be discharged from theatres to Ward A.

Next text cycle

Plan: Trial the guideline on the first three patients transferred to Ward A by the participating surgeons on the next Tuesday. Nurse practitioner J to make sure that the guideline is available on the ward and talk to as many staff as possible about the trial. Nurse practitioner J will interview the nurses who use the guideline to find out if they had found the guideline easy to use.

Do: The guideline was trialled on two patients.

Study: One of the patients was missed from the trial because the member of nursing staff looking after the patient was not aware of the project and therefore was not aware of the guideline. Results showed that both of the patients included in the trial showed improvements in symptoms after receiving the fluid. The time between nurse assessment of deterioration and the bolus of fluid being given was 30 minutes for both patients. Both the nurses interviewed after the trial said that they were nervous about the new responsibility but the guideline had been easy to read and use.

Act: Continue the trial on orthopaedic patients discharged to Ward A next week. Set up a project storyboard at the entrance to the ward and ask the senior sister on ward A to brief all her staff, including part-time and night staff about the project.

Throughout the project nursing staff on the wards were asked to collect details on the time they assessed the patient and the time the patient received their fluid. This time to be plotted on a chart on the wall of the ward to keep track of their progress. Over the two month period of the trial the run chart was created as shown in Figure 12.8.

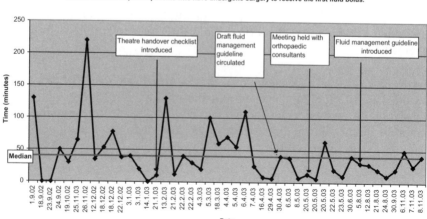

Figure 12.8 Fluid management final run chart.

Early results showed that the changes implemented on the ward had reduced the delay in administering fluid to patients after surgery. The ward staff found the method of data collection easy and were motivated to make suggestions for new change ideas as a result of seeing the chart on the wall developing over time. The decision was made to continue to collect and display the data in the same way to monitor the sustainability of the project.

The outreach team asked some of the staff from the orthopaedic ward to present their results at the next link nurse meeting in the hope that other wards would adopt similar practice. They hoped that the spread of ideas would achieve their overall aim to reduce the total number of calls they received for patients needing fluid.

REFERENCES

Bens I (2000) *Facilitating with Ease: A Step by Step Guidebook with Customizable Worksheets on CD-Rom*. Jossey Bass.

Berwick DM (2003) Disseminating innovations in healthcare. *Journal of the American Medical Assocation* 289: 1969–75.

Department of Health (2005) NHS Modernisation Agency. *Improvement Leaders' Guides*. London: Department of Health.

Fraser SW (2002) *Accelerating the Spread of Good Practice: A Workbook for Healthcare*. Chichester: Kingsham Press.

Goal/QPC (1995) *Coach's Guide to the Memory Jogger II*. Salem, NH: Goal/QPC.

Iles V, Sutherland K (2001) *Managing Change in the NHS: Organisational Change*. London: NCCSDO.

Institute for Healthcare Improvement (2005) *Information Gathering Tools*. Boston, MA: Institute for Healthcare Improvement. http://www.QualityHealthCare.org

Langley GJ, Nolan KM, Nolan TW, Norman CL, Provost, LP (1996) *The Improvement Guide. A Practical Approach to Enhancing Organizational Performance*. San Francisco: Jossey-Bass.

Plesk PE (1999) Section 1: Evidence-based quality improvement, principles and perspectives. *Quality Improvement Methods in Clinical Medicine* 13(1): 203–14.

Rainey TG, Kabcenell A, Berwick D, Roessner J (1998) *Reducing Costs and Improving Outcomes in Adult Intensive Care*. Breakthrough Series Guide. Boston: Institute for Healthcare Improvement.

FURTHER READING

Beckhard R, Harris R (1987) *Organisational Transitions: Managing Complex Change*. Addison Wesley OD Series.

Department of Health (2004) NHS Modernisation Agency. *10 High Impact Changes for Service Improvement and Delivery*. London: Department of Health.

Silversin J, Kornacki MJ (2000) *Leading Physicians through Change: How to Achieve and Sustain Results*. Florida: American College of Physician Executives.

13 Evaluation of critical care outreach: are the resources for outreach justified?

PAUL WHITING AND DAVID EDBROOKE

INTRODUCTION

The concept of outreach is relatively recent and its development has been addressed in other chapters of this book. The concept embraces the idea that by identifying patients who are deteriorating on the ward they can be either treated appropriately on the ward or referred early for critical care admission. Much work has been seen in this area over the past few years and it is important to ask whether care has been improved through the establishment of outreach teams. This chapter considers this question and in doing so gives an overview of evaluative work undertaken so far.

In the United Kingdom many outreach teams were initiated in response to requests for this service by the Department of Health in 2000. This followed the publication of a comprehensive review of critical care services (DoH 2000) in which it was indicated that outreach care was required for three reasons:

1. to avert admissions by helping prevent further deterioration or ensuring admission to critical care in a timely fashion;
2. to enable discharges by supporting patients who have been discharged to the wards;
3. to share critical care skills with other staff in other hospital areas.

NHS trusts were subsequently invited to bid for funding, from the newly formed critical care networks, to establish and develop critical care outreach teams (Priestly et al. 2004). The drive for the implementation of outreach services has continued with the full support of the Secretary of State who in 2003 wrote that 'we should see outreach services developing in every hospital' (Modernisation Agency 2003).

Critical Care Outreach. Edited by Lee Cutler and Wayne Robson.
Copyright 2006 by John Wiley & Sons Ltd.

At the time of introduction no large-scale evaluations had been undertaken to ascertain the benefits that might accrue from introducing the concept. In addition no evidence-based guidelines were available about how many staff should be devoted to outreach, what skill level was required, whether it should be physicians, nurses, physiotherapist or a mixture of all. Finally no information was available as to whether the service should be available in office hours or on a 24-hours-a-day, 7-days-a-week basis. This led to varying models of outreach being adopted nationally. Each individual Trust developed a model in line with its available resources and perceived service requirement (Richardson et al. 2004).

The differences in the staffing of teams, models and actual service dynamics that subsequently developed meant no two services were identical. This national variation, along with the haste in which the services were developed and implemented, means that evaluation is not simple.

To undertake an evaluation of this type is time-consuming and difficult. It has the same problems as other critical care trials in that there are numerous confounding factors. These are mainly due to the wide variation in diagnoses, chronic health status, and the quality of care received within the critical care and ward environments. Consequently, to achieve a statistically significant difference in any two groups of critical care patients will require the enrolment of many thousands of patients. This is reflected in the patient numbers recruited in almost all critical care trials that examined the differences between groups (Knaus et al. 1985, 1986, 1989; Gall et al. 1993). In addition to this, the costs of conducting such trials are high. Perhaps for all these reasons a large evaluation has not been undertaken though with the introduction of more outreach services and the expansion of existing ones, an evaluation seems ever more necessary. However, such evaluation would not be without its difficulties and the outcomes from future and ongoing evaluations are eagerly awaited by the critical care community.

There are some parallels with intensive care, which emerged in the 1950s without any evaluations to prove its benefits when compared to other traditional care models. Fifty years on it would seem unlikely that any ethical committee would agree to randomising 50% of patients judged to require intensive care, not to receive it. While the case is not quite as dramatic with regards to outreach, it is perhaps unlikely that ethical committees would agree to randomisation of care to include or exclude established outreach care.

EVALUATION

To address the question of whether the resources put into outreach have so far been justified, we must appreciate that no one model for outreach has been adopted within the UK (Richardson et al. 2004). We can therefore only address the question of justification by looking at all of outreach's individual components, such as ward staff education, patient follow-up and identification of the sick ward patient.

Difficulties in evaluation can also arise when one considers the clinicians' interpretation of such things as quality of care and the appropriateness and timeliness of ICU admission, as these can and do vary enormously (Groom et al. 2001). Equally, the concept of sub-optimal care is ill defined and based upon subjective opinion, often influenced by an individual's experience and knowledge.

The national perspective (Modernisation Agency 2003) is that the evaluation of outreach services involves the following parameters.

• Reduction in number of 'unexpected' cardiac arrest calls

It was shown that after the introduction of a medical emergency team in Australia, the incidence of cardiac arrest was reduced (Story et al. 2004). Early warning scores and subsequent patient referrals have also shown a decrease in the number of, but not the overall mortality from, cardiopulmonary arrest. It was argued that this was because the potentially salvageable cases had been prevented from progressing to an irretrievable clinical condition (Lee et al. 1995).

• Facilitated DNARs

There is emerging evidence of a consistent and measurable impact of early warning scoring and the role of the outreach team in timely Do Not Attempt Resuscitation decision-making (Morgan 2003). This not only allows for a timely and dignified death in appropriate circumstances but also reduces the frequency of protracted and often inappropriate use of resources.

• Reduction in re-admissions

Outreach has been shown to enable follow-up of post-critical care patients helping prevent re-admission to those potentially discharged inappropriately or too early from ICU (Goldfrad and Rowan 2000; Leary and Ridley 2003). This is important and significant as re-admitted patients have a sevenfold increase in mortality when compared with those who have not been discharged too soon (Leary and Ridley 2003). Other studies have noted that outreach has had no impact upon the number of critical care re-admissions, but has decreased the number of unexpected admissions (Brown 2003; Leary and Ridley 2003).

• Averted critical care admissions

Audits have highlighted a statistically significant reduction (p = 0.05) in the emergency admission rate to ICU, on those wards covered by outreach teams, during the hours of 09.00–17.00. Although their subsequent stay was shorter, this was clinically rather than statistically significant (Pittard 2003).

• **Reduction in overall hospital mortality**
Outreach and its interventions have been shown to reduce the admission **A**cute **P**hysiology **A**nd **C**hronic **H**ealth **E**valuation (APACHE) scores so helping to improve critical care and hospital mortality (Modernisation Agency 2003). They have also helped to significantly ($p = 0.05$) reduce the mortality rates on those wards they have covered (Pittard 2003).

• **Timing of referrals**
Overall the effect of outreach and the early warning scoring systems has been to alert the medical staff and critical care physicians to the worsening physiological parameters of the patient, so enabling earlier and appropriate medical intervention (Stenhouse et al. 2000). Not only is the score itself very useful but also the frequency of scoring, as this allows the outreach team to assess improvement or deterioration following an intervention. This has been shown to help avert subsequent admission to critical care (Pittard 2003). Once the physiological variables are abnormal and the patient identified, outreach has been shown to reduce the delay in admission to critical care, and the time spent on the emergency admissions unit (Modernisation Agency 2003).

• **Improvement in recording of variables**
It has been proven that greater than 50% of ward patients who develop an acute critical illness show signs of deterioration over many hours prior to their admission to critical care (Bamgbade 2002). The calculation of the early warning scores, an integral part of outreach, helps ensure that all variables are measured and subsequently acted upon. Yet, in the recent MERIT (**M**edical **E**arly **R**esponse, **I**ntervention and **T**herapy) study, one of the conclusions drawn was that a large number of adverse events had occurred without the recording of vital signs, a contradiction to other authors' experiences (Hillman 2005).

Advancements in critical care and anaesthetic techniques have enabled higher risk patients to undergo major surgical procedures that would have previously been inappropriate. These patients are often older and acutely unwell increasing the acuity and dependency of the patients on acute general wards (McCarthur-Rouse 2001). The most important factor in the improvement of post-operative care is to define and then enhance the role of the nursing staff. Empowering them to take therapeutic measures will avoid the delay and indecision of inexperienced junior doctors that contribute to morbidity and mortality (Wunsch et al. 2004). This is best done through education, although there is a lack of evidence as to how exactly this is best achieved (McCarthur-Rouse 2001).

THE COSTS OF OUTREACH

The development of outreach within any hospital should not be seen as a cost effective substitute for the insufficient provision of critical care beds, poor ward facilities or inadequate staffing.

• Staff

The most common group of staff undertaking outreach care are nurses. They are usually very experienced and thus consume significant resources because of their senior clinical grade. Ideally the service should be available 24 hours per day and 365 days per year (DoH 2005; NCEPOD 2005) but resources are not generally available for this level of service. Therefore most outreach services are only available during routine office hours. This is perhaps inappropriate as a lot of referrals, more than 50%, occur between 2100 hours and 0800 hours and at weekends (Barnett et al. 2002; Wunsch et al. 2004) when outreach staff are not available.

The Medical Economics and Research Centre, Sheffield (MERCS) routinely audit approximately 80 ICUs throughout the UK in the United Kingdom Cost Block Programme (Edbrooke et al. 1999). Data from this audit is useful in giving an indication of the relative costs of staff in outreach (The Cost Block Programme Appendix 13.1). While outreach is a hospital-wide service it is usually funded through critical care budgets and so is presented here as cost per ICU bed.

It is as yet unclear what skill mix is appropriate, but nurse consultants and other senior grades are the commonest with some trusts employing physiotherapists in this role. The mean annual nursing and physiotherapy cost of outreach (per ICU bed) for 2003/04 is shown in Table 13.1. However, there is a large variation in costs and provision with annual cost per ICU bed varying regionally between £1931 and £7301

These costs equate to a mean cost of £15.9 per patient day. This accounts for 1.5% of the daily cost per patient; consequently we can conclude that this is a low-cost initiative.

Medical staff are also utilised within outreach, both in sessions for patient review and for teaching. From the cost block report for 2003–4 based on 81 ICUs, the mean annual cost per ICU bed is £456. Table 13.2 gives comparative annual costs for nursing, consultant medical staff and physiotherapy in outreach. It can be seen that consultant medical staff are a small fraction of the cost of the total service.

• Resources other than staff

Most hospitals have developed a form with which to chart early warning signs of patient deterioration. Usually these have been developed and piloted over a long period of time and consequently are a cost to the hospital. No figures

Table 13.1 Mean annual cost of outreach (per ICU bed)

Physiotherapy	£85.00
Nurse consultants	£705.30
Established nurses	£3636.90
Totals	**£4427.20**

Table 13.2 The mean annual cost of outreach (£) (2003/04)

	Consultant cost	Nursing cost	Physiotherapy cost
Number of ICUs	77	80	80
Mean cost	£4,312.30	£45,007.04	£785.12
SD	£13,771.00	£54,993.57	£3,829.20

are available but while it is unrealistic to say that the costs are zero, as the staff are already employed, they could be viewed as an opportunity cost (Hillman et al. 2003). This implies that by doing this task the opportunity for them to undertake other tasks is lost.

• Teaching

The costs and the time involved in supporting and educating ward staff are unknown, but undoubtedly required (McCarthur-Rouse 2001). Staff will have to be released from the ward environment for a period of time, constituting a cost in staff time. To the authors' knowledge there is no data on the resources required and hence the cost but it is clear that compared to the costs of ICU it is small.

• Savings

While some of the costs and resources that are required to operate an outreach service are partially measurable, and seemingly quite small, the benefits are deemed to be beneficial but unproven. It is a pity that outreach was not developed in a more structured way beginning with a multi-centre trial comparing hospitals or wards that had an outreach service with those that did not. The disadvantages are that it would be time-consuming and expensive. However, from these data could be gleaned effectiveness, and if the costs of the two arms of the trial were also known the incremental cost effectiveness ratio could therefore be calculated. This simply means the differences in effectiveness divided by the differences in cost.

At this stage it would appear unlikely that this will be undertaken in the near future and we can only speculate as to whether an outreach service is cost effective. However, it would seem a reasonable view that comparing the small costs of providing the service to the very high cost of intensive care then it appears very likely that it is a cost-effective service. From the information above the saving in ICU costs would only have to exceed 1.5% of the cost per patient day, for this to be the case.

EFFECTIVENESS

As previously discussed, the question as to whether the investment in outreach services has been justified is a difficult one, due in part to its lack of preceding evidence base and few international equivalents to act as a benchmark. The Australian equivalent, the Medical Emergency Teams (METs), have recently undergone a randomised controlled evaluation (Hillman 2005) in which the conclusions were disappointing. Despite their increased utilisation during the study period, they failed to substantially affect the incidence of cardiac arrest, unplanned ICU admission or unexpected death. A large number of adverse events had also occurred without the documenting of vital signs and, more worryingly, when they were documented there were numerous occasions when no action was taken.

These recent findings from a large randomised controlled trial are in contrast to other lower grades of evidence that support the role of outreach. These highlight the significantly reduced readmission rates, some by greater than 50%, to ICU (Modernisation Agency 2003), improved survival to discharge (Ball et al. 2003; Hillman 2003) and ICU mortality (Pittard 2003). Yet other authors have contradicted this stating little proven benefit, especially no effect on mortality (Bristow 2000).

In view of this one would expect a shorter length of hospital stay and hence recovery. But some authors have suggested that outreach interventions actually increase patients' length of hospital stay (Priestly et al. 2004), despite the fact that one study has demonstrated a decrease in the average length of ICU stay from 7.4 to 4.8 days (Pittard 2003). This may be in part due to the earlier recognition and lower admission APACHE scores of patients (Modernisation Agency 2003), and the survival of those patients who may not have otherwise survived without outreach intervention.

Quality of life has been defined as 'a patient's appraisal of and satisfaction with their current level of functioning as compared to what they perceive to be possible or ideal' (Cella and Tulsky 1990). Outreach's effect upon quality of life for a patient is difficult to assess. Nevertheless it is important to consider that prolonged ventilation and stay on ICU is associated with an impaired health-related quality of life compared with that of a matched general population (Combes et al. 2003). Outreach could theoretically influence a patient's post-ICU quality of life by shortening the duration of ICU therapy and stay. Not only is this significant to the patient but also to society since productivity, post-critical illness, may increase.

BALANCED EVALUATION

Answering questions about the effectiveness of critical care outreach requires that services are evaluated. Service evaluation has been defined as:

A set of procedures to judge a service's merit by providing a systematic assessment of its aims, objectives, activities outputs, outcomes and costs. (NHS Executive 1997)

This may involve research methods as well as clinical audit. Searching the published literature highlights that relatively little research has been undertaken to evaluate critical care outreach. While not all research undertaken is subsequently published, the professional literature gives a guide as to the extent of investigation. Much of the work undertaken to date might more correctly be called 'audit'. It is important to understand the differences between research and audit and most importantly to understand how valuable audit can be in enhancing our understanding of critical care outreach and the care of the seriously ill outside of the ICU/HDU environment.

Research and audit are different but interrelated activities (Hardman and Joughin 1998). Their relationship is that they support and inform each other but are different in their aims and outcomes, though some of the methods employed in the process may be shared.

Some important points that help differentiate audit and research are included here and have been adapted from Hardman and Joughin (1998).

- Research aims to establish what best practice is, while audit aims to evaluate how close practice is to standards that may have been set as a result of research.
- Research is designed so that it can be replicated and its results generalised to other similar groups, whereas audit is specific and local to one patient group or one setting and hence not generalisable.
- Research aims to generate new knowledge or increase the sum of knowledge, whereas audit aims to improve services. Thus research is theory driven, whereas audit is practice based.
- Research may be a single study, whereas audit is an ongoing process.

This final point highlights the cyclical nature of audit, where standard setting, review of adherence to standards, changes in practice and standards, and re-audit are key features. Audit can evaluate *structure, process* and *outcome* (Donabedian 1966); these are important areas to consider in critical care outreach since outreach teams vary so much in this regard. The resources allocated (structure) and the model of intervention versus education and advice (process) vary so significantly within the field that outcomes may well vary.

Much can be learned through sharing of clinical audit findings and many very useful answers to important questions can be obtained with the outcomes of improving practice and systems. While the critical care community eagerly awaits the results of future research and reviews of outreach, the role of other methods of evaluation and the accumulation of understanding that can be gained through these activities when shared and critically debated in professional forums should be acknowledged.

In a case study which follows Chapter 2, Dr David Wood has shared a useful audit he undertook regarding the best way to employ a track and trigger system.

A final point on balanced evaluation is to acknowledge the value of qualitative data and qualitative methods in evaluation (Murphy et al. 1998). While there is considerable interest in answering the question 'Does outreach reduce mortality and morbidity?', it is important to view health outcomes in a more holistic way. Such outcomes for outreach might include, for example, the way that outreach has affected the culture of critical care in acute ward areas and the way that this culture in turn affects the care of the critically ill. A further important issue is the contribution that outreach makes to the patient experience of critical illness and the way patients are cared for when they are frightened, vulnerable and disorientated. These areas are conspicuously absent in the research literature regarding critical care outreach and they pose an interesting and worthwhile challenge to future researchers in this area.

THE WAY AHEAD

In view of the recent MERIT trial results the withdrawal of a medical emergency team or outreach service may appear to be justified (Hillman 2005). This would be unlikely as many of the nursing and junior medical staff have become so used to the educational, practical and advisory support offered by outreach, that they would probably not allow the service to be withdrawn (Hillman et al. 2003). Considering critical care in general 'while there is a strong database about the illnesses of patients, there has been a dearth of useful management information about critical care resources, the treatments given and their effectiveness' (Audit Commission 1999, p. 3).

What is known has taken years to build and in some instances gives a clear indication of the benefits that can be gained from critical care intervention. The implications for outreach are that understanding will become more sophisticated as we learn why research so far has delivered mixed results.

Will the outreach team, as we know it, continue to function in a similar manner in the future? Several authors have proposed differing approaches to providing 24 hour, seven days a week cover within the current financial and staffing constraints. These include combining the role of the acute pain team and outreach so integrating skills and providing an increased level of cover (Counsell 2001), developing the role of the night nurse practitioner (Riley and Falerio 2004), and the formation of specific perioperative care teams in place of outreach (Bamgbade 2002).

In summary the role of outreach will undoubtedly evolve and develop, and the question as to whether its resource allocation has been, or in the future will be, justified is difficult to say. We can only continue to evaluate its key components ensuring their effectiveness and evolution in the context of changing needs and the ever-increasing demands placed upon it.

REFERENCES

Audit Commission (1999) *Critical to Success: The Place of Efficient and Effective Critical Care Services within the Acute Hospital.* London: Audit Commission.

Ball C, Kirkby M, Williams S (2003) Effect of the critical care outreach team on patient survival to discharge from hospital and readmission to critical care: non-randomised population based study. *British Medical Journal* 327(7422).

Bamgbade O (2002) The peri-operative care team: a model for outreach critical care. *Anaesthesia* 57: 1028–9.

Barnett MJ, Kaboli PJ, Sirio CA, Rosenthal GE (2002) Day of the week of intensive care unit admission and patient outcomes: a multisite regional evaluation. *Medical Care* 40(6): 530–9.

Bristow PJ (2000) Rate of hospital arrest, deaths and intensive care admissions: the effect of the medical emergency team. *Medical Journal of Australia* 173: 236–40.

Brown J (2003) Response to the impact of outreach team on re-admission to a critical care unit. *Anaesthesia* 58: 828.

Cella DF, Tulsky DS (1990) Measuring quality of life today: methodological aspects. *Oncology* 4: 29–38.

Combes A, Costa MA, Trouillet JL et al. (2003) Morbidity, mortality, and quality of life outcomes of patients requiring > 14 days of mechanical ventilation. *Critical Care Medicine* 31(5): 1378–81.

Counsell D (2001) The acute pain service: a model for outreach critical care. *Anaesthesia* 56: 925–6.

Department of Health (2000) *Comprehensive Critical Care: A Review of Adult Critical Care Services.* London: Department of Health.

Department of Health (2005) *Quality Critical Care: Beyond 'Comprehensive Critical Care'. A Report by the Stakeholder Forum.* London: Department of Health.

Donabedian A (1966) Evaluating the quality of medical care. *Millbank Memorial Federation of Quality* 44: 166–208.

Edbrooke D, Hibbert C, Ridley S et al. (1999) The development of a method for comparative costing of individual intensive care units: the intensive care working group on costing. *Anaesthesia* 54(2): 110–20.

Gall JRL, Lemeshow S, Sulnier F (1993) A new simplified acute physiology score (SAPS II) based on a European/North American multicenter study. *JAMA* 270: 2957–63.

Goldfrad C, Rowan K (2000) Consequences of discharges from intensive care at night. *Lancet* 355: 1138–42.

Groom P, Neary H, Wellbeloved S (2001) Critical care without walls: the outreach experience of one Trust (Part 2). *Nursing in Critical Care* 6(6): 279–84.

Hardman E, Joughin C (1998) *Focus on Clinical Audit. Child and Adolescent Mental Health Services*. London: Royal Colleges of Psychiatrists.

Hillman K (2003) Correspondence to outreach critical care. *British Journal of Anaesthesia* 90(6): 808.

Hillman K (2005) Introduction of the medical emergency team (MET) system: a cluster randomised controlled trial. *Lancet* 365: 2091–7.

Hillman K, Chen J, Brown D (2003) A clinical model for health services research – the medical emergency team. *Journal of Critical Care* 18(1): 195–9.

Knaus WA, Draper EA, Wagner D, Zimmerman JE (1985) APACHE II: A severity of disease classification system. *Critical Care Medicine* 13: 818–29.

Knaus WA, Draper EA, Wagner DP, Zimmerman JE (1986) An evaluation of outcome from intensive care in major medical centres. *Annals of Internal Medicine* 104(3): 410–18.

Knaus WA, Wagner DP, Draper EA (1989) APACHE III study design: analytic plan for evaluation of severity of outcome in intensive care unit patients: Implications. *Critical Care Medicine* 17(12 part 2): S219–21.

Leary T, Ridley S (2003) Impact of outreach on re-admission to a critical care unit. *Anaesthesia* 58: 328–32.

Lee A, Bishop G, Hillman K, Daffurn K (1995) The medical emergency team. *Anaesthesia and Intensive Care* 23: 183–6.

McCarthur-Rouse F (2001) Critical care outreach services and early warning scoring systems: a review of the literature. *Journal of Advanced Nursing* 36(5): 696–704.

Modernisation Agency (2003) *The National Outreach Report 2003: Progress in Developing Services*. London: Department of Health and Modernisation Agency.

Morgan RJ (2003) Outreach critical care – cash for no questions. *British Journal of Anaesthesia* 90(5): 700.

Murphy E, Dingwall R, Greatbatch D, Parker S, Watson P (1998) Qualitative research methods in health technology assessment: a review of the literature. *Health Technology Assessment* 2(16).

National Health Service Executive (1997) *Personal Medical Services. Pilots under the NHS. A Guide to Local Evaluation*. London: Department of Health.

NCEPOD (2005) '*An Acute Problem?*' London: National Confidential Enquiry into Patient Outcomes and Death.

Pittard AJ (2003) Out of our reach? Assessing the impact of introducing a critical care outreach service. *Anaesthesia* 58(9): 882–5.

Priestly G, Watson W, Rashidian A et al. (2004) Introducing critical care outreach: a ward randomised trial of phased introduction in a general hospital. *Intensive Care Medicine* 30: 1398–1404.

Richardson A, Burnard V, Colley H, Coulter C (2004) Ward nurses' evaluation of critical care outreach. *Nursing in Critical Care* 9(1): 28–33.

Riley B, Falerio R (2001) Critical care outreach: rationale and development. *British Journal of Anaesthesia* 1: 146–9.

Stenhouse C, Coates S, Tivey M et al. (2000) Prospective valuation of a modified early warning score to aid earlier detection of patients developing critical illness on a surgical ward. *British Journal of Anaesthesia* 84: 663.

Story D, Shelton A, Poustie S et al. (2004) The effect of critical care outreach on postoperative serious adverse events. *Anaesthesia* 59: 762–6.

Wunsch H, Mapstone J, Brady T et al. (2004) Hospital mortality associated with day and time of admission to intensive care units. *Intensive Care Medicine* 30(5): 895–901.

APPENDIX 13.1

The cost block programme measures top down costs. This means that the total cost of an ICU is calculated from various groups of costs. It is retrospective as the costs are collected after the time period, usually a financial year. In its development by a multi-disciplinary group including clinicians and economists, six groups or blocks of cost were identified:

• capital equipment
• estates (the fabric of the building)
• non-clinical support costs (management and infrastructure)
• clinical support costs (physiotherapy, laboratory services)
• consumables (drugs and disposables)
• staff.

Two pilot trials were undertaken and it was clear that the first three cost blocks were difficult to collect and consistently accounted for only 15% of the total costs. Thus they were removed from further data collections and the system was launched nationally in 1998–9.

Since then it has been internally validated extensively and work as yet unpublished shows good internal consistency of data returns.

Index

Critical Care Outreach. Edited by Lee Cutler and Wayne Robson.
Copyright 2006 by John Wiley & Sons Ltd.